NONVERBAL LEARNING DISABILITIES

Nonverbal Learning Disabilities
The Syndrome and the Model

BYRON P. ROURKE
University of Windsor

THE GUILFORD PRESS
New York   London

© 1989 The Guilford Press
A Division of Guilford Publications, Inc.
72 Spring Street, New York, NY 10012

Printed in the United States of America

Last digit is print number: 9 8 7 6 5 4

Library of Congress Cataloging-in-Publication Data
Rourke, Byron P. (Byron Patrick), 1939–
    Nonverbal learning disabilities: the syndrome and the model/
Byron P. Rourke.
        p.   cm.
    Bibliography: p.
    Includes index.
    ISBN 0-89862-378-2
    1. Learning disabilities.   I. Title.
RJ506.L4R68   1989
618.92′89—dc 19   89-1958
                                                          CIP

In the late 1940s and early 1950s, Ralph M. Reitan launched a research program that revolutionized the manner in which the scientific and clinical aspects of human neuropsychology were to transpire for the next 40 years. In 1975, Helmer R. Myklebust published a chapter, entitled "Nonverbal Learning Disabilities," that has had a profound effect on the direction of our research program. In 1981, Elkhonon Goldberg and Louis Costa published a landmark theoretical paper that has formed the basis of my theoretical and model-building activities since that time. Without the seminal works of these scientists, the present work would never have seen the light of day. For these and other reasons too numerous to mention, this book is, with affection, dedicated to the four of them—whether they like it or not.

Acknowledgments

This book could not have been written without the scientific and clinical contributions of several of my colleagues, former students, and current students. In this respect, I would acknowledge in particular the thoughtful contributions to my thinking about nonverbal learning disabilities by those with whom I have worked most closely. They include Gerald C. Young, M. Alan J. Finlayson, John L. Fisk, Jerel E. Del Dotto, John D. Strang, Rhea Finnell, John E. DeLuca, Diane L. Russell, and Edite J. Ozols. Others whose comments and reviews have been particularly helpful include Joseph E. Casey, Mary L. Stewart, Joanna Hamilton, Clare Brandys, and Kenneth M. Adams. Sara Sparrow, Jerel E. Del Dotto, Domenic V. Cicchetti, and Harry van der Vlugt read the entire text and offered very helpful comments on it. The Herculean efforts of Sean B. Rourke in bringing this book to fruition are gratefully acknowledged, as are the perspicacious comments on the text by Marilyn F. Chedour. Finally, although it may go without saying, I should state for the record that any inadequacies that remain in this work are, of course, my responsibility.

Preface

The present work was designed to describe and explain the elements and dynamics of the nonverbal learning disability (NLD) syndrome and of the NLD model. Furthermore, an attempt is made to deal with the ramifications of the NLD syndrome and model in the theoretical and applied aspects of the neuropsychology of learning disabilities and in the general field of child clinical neuropsychology.

Chapter 1 provides background information, while Chapter 2 contains reasonably detailed explanations of several approaches that we have employed in an effort to determine the neuropsychological characteristics of various subtypes of learning-disabled children. Chapter 3 deals with one important aspect of investigative efforts in this area, namely, the socioemotional disturbances of learning-disabled children. These chapters serve as a kind of prolegomena to those that follow, all of which are devoted to an examination of the NLD syndrome. Chapter 4 contains a description of the Rourke (1982) model. Focusing on differences between right- and left-hemisphere functioning, this model was designed to encompass and explain many of the research findings in the neuropsychology of learning disabilities that are contained in Chapters 2 and 3. The NLD syndrome and model are described in detail in Chapters 5 and 6, the latter also containing generalizations derived from the NLD model that relate to various theoretical and clinical issues in the field of child clinical neuropsychology. In order to illustrate the clinical implications of this syndrome, a number of issues are addressed in Chapter 7. This chapter also contains detailed descriptions of the comprehensive neuropsychological examinations of several children and adolescents who manifest the NLD syndrome. The work concludes with Chapter 8, which is essentially a postscript dealing with some of the implications of the NLD syndrome and model for definitions of learning disabilities and for future investigative efforts within this area of scientific endeavor.

One final note: The description of research that has emanated from our laboratory, as presented in Chapter 2 and sections of Chapter 3, is designed to coincide roughly with the stages of the development of the NLD model and with the developmental progression of its manifestations in children. This was done so that the reader might share in the process of discovery that my colleagues and I have found so intensely captivating and intriguing.

Contents

NONVERBAL LEARNING DISABILITIES

CHAPTER ONE

Introduction

This book is about an odyssey of research and clinical efforts that has culminated in the isolation of a pattern of neuropsychological abilities and deficits characterized as the nonverbal learning disabilities (NLD) syndrome. This investigative journey began in the late 1960s, with publications describing this work appearing in the early 1970s. To convey the full impact of the NLD syndrome within the field of the neuropsychology of learning disabilities and, more generally, within the scientific and applied aspects of child clinical neuropsychology, I felt it was necessary to describe in some detail how my colleagues and I have worked on this investigative project over the past 20 years.

Before doing so, however, it would be well to address two topics in this introductory chapter. First, this research effort needs to be placed within the historical context of the study of learning disabilities in children, specifically, within the context of the study of learning disability subtypes, of which the NLD syndrome is one. Second, it is necessary to describe in some detail the systematic developmental neuropsychological approach to the study of learning disabilities in children that has guided our research efforts in this area, as well as how this approach has evolved as a result of our work.

THE HISTORICAL CONTEXT

Learning Disabilities as a Homogeneous Entity

There is an important similarity between the history of the neuropsychological study of learning disabilities in children and the investigation of frankly brain-damaged individuals. This lies in the fact that most early investigators in both of these areas of scientific endeavor subscribed to a particular viewpoint, one that managed to hold sway for a protracted period of time during the development of these fields. It held that impaired individuals (be they learning disabled or brain damaged) have very much in common with others who are so afflicted. This led investigators to maintain, either explicitly or implicitly, that there was such a unitary entity as the "brain-damaged child" or the "learning-disabled child." In turn, they felt that significant advances in our understanding of the neuropsychological dimensions of these disorders would be derived from studies that involved comparisons of children suffering from either of these two types of disorder with appropriately matched controls (i.e., normal children) on carefully selected variables of theoretical interest.

As can be gleaned from any systematic review of the learning-disabilities literature prior to the late 1970s (e.g., Benton, 1975; Rourke, 1978a), this "comparative-populations" (Applebee, 1971) or "contrasting-groups" investigative strategy was the approach adopted almost exclusively by North American and European researchers. Studies involving comparisons of groups of supposedly learning-disabled youngsters with groups of "normal" controls, matched for age and other factors, were employed to determine *the* abilities and deficits that characterize the neuropsychological ability structure of *the* learning-disabled child (Doehring, 1978). The use of this method for the determination of the neuropsychological abilities and deficits of learning-disabled children assumed, implicitly or explicitly, that such children formed an univocal, homogeneous diagnostic entity.

This approach was also characterized by rather narrow samplings of areas of human performance that were thought to be related to the learning (primarily reading) disability. For example, some researchers who were convinced that a deficiency in memory formed the basis for learning disabilities in youngsters would follow the rather straightforward research tack of measuring and comparing "memory" in groups of learning-disabled children and their matched controls. Almost without fail, the conclusion of such a research effort was that learning-disabled children were deficient in memory and that it was this deficient memory that was the cause of their learning disability. Indeed, the only crucial variable that would influence the results of such studies was the severity of the learning deficit of the learning-disabled subjects studied: The more severe the learning deficit, the more likely it was that the contrasting groups would differ.

Such research was periodically seen as somewhat shortsighted and inconclusive, because it could be demonstrated, for example, that disabled learners were more deficient in "auditory memory" than they were in "visual memory." This constituted something of an advance in the field, since a rather more comprehensive sampling of skills and abilities was undertaken in this sort of study. However, there remained the commitment to the contrasting-groups methodology, and there was one other complicating factor that crept into the considerations of investigators in the field. This could best be described as the developmental dimension. Specifically, it became clear to some that one "obtained" significant differences between contrasting groups of disabled and normal readers on some variables and not on others as an apparent function of the age at which the children were studied. Thus, an example of the next advance that took place in this research tradition was to compare groups of younger and older children on auditory and visual memory tasks to determine if the main effects (for auditory and visual memory) and the interactions (with age) were significant.

Even with these advances, however, there remained the reluctance of those who adopted this essentially narrow, nomothetic approach to engage in the analysis of the abilities and deficits of individual learning-disabled children. For example, it was rarely the case that investigators would report results of individual cases in their studies of auditory and visual memory, even though this is very simply accomplished (see Czudner & Rourke, 1972, and Rourke & Czudner, 1972, for examples of how individual results can be reported in such studies). Thus, we have been left with group results that may not reflect how all individuals within the group performed. Some critics of this nomothetic approach to the understanding of learning disabilities in children adopted a position that was quite antithetical to it, one that is best described as an "idiographic" or "idiosyncratic" approach to the field.

Learning Disabilities as an Idiographic Disorder

As was the case in the history of the study of frank brain damage in youngsters, there have been investigators in the field of learning disabilities who would maintain that persons so designated exhibit unique, idiographic, nongeneralizable origins, characteristics, and reactions to their afflictions and, as such, must be treated on an individual basis. Investigators of this ilk would suggest that the single-case study is the only viable means for discovering valid scientific information. They would also argue that the important dimensions of this disorder are individualized to the extent that meaningful generalizations are virtually impossible.

It is clear that this point of view contrasts sharply and in almost all respects with the contrasting-groups position outlined. This nomothetic/idiographic debate is not unique to the study of learning disabilities and frankly brain-damaged individuals. (A particularly poignant and insightful characterization of this nomothetic/idiographic controversy in the entire field of clinical neuropsychology has been presented by Reitan, 1974.)

Critique of the Contrasting-Groups and Idiographic Approaches

Contrasting-Groups Approach

As suggested earlier, studies within this tradition served to do little more than produce a lengthy catalogue of variables that differentiate "learning-disabled" from "normal" children (Rourke, 1978a). Considered as a whole, the results of this corpus of research made it abundantly evident that virtually any single measure of perceptual, psycholinguistic, or higher-order cognitive skill could be used to illustrate the superiority of normal children over comparable groups of children diagnosed as learning disabled.

There are many who still persist in comparative-populations or contrasting-groups methodology, however, with all of the limitations that it involves, with respect not only to research findings but to model building and theory development. This mode of approach to research has not contributed a great deal. The results of many studies are trivial, contradictory to one another, and not supported in replication attempts; further, there is little to suggest that the factors identified as "characteristic" of learning-disabled children in these studies are related to one another in any meaningful fashion (Rourke, 1985). In sum, the evidence regarding cognitive, mnestic, and other forms of functioning that emerges from the contrasting-groups approach to research is, at best, equivocal. A coherent and meaningful pattern of neuropsychological characteristics of children with learning disabilities does not emerge from this literature. I would maintain that this is the case because the assumption of a univocal pattern upon which it is based does not obtain. (I will say more on this point shortly.)

In any event, there would appear to be at least three major reasons why the results of these studies have not contributed much to the testing of important hypotheses relating to the neuropsychological integrity of learning-disabled youngsters. These, together with some brief comments on alternative approaches, are as follows:

1. Lack of a Conceptual Model. In the vast majority of studies that can be characterized in terms of the comparative-populations or contrasting-groups rubric, there is an obvious absence of a comprehensive conceptual model that could be employed to elucidate the skills involved in perception, learning, memory, and cognition, which are deficient in learning-disabled children. Most models that have been developed in this genre of research bear the marks of either post-hoc theorizing about a very limited spectrum of skills and abilities or "pet" theories derived from what are characterized as more "general" models of perception, learning, memory, and cognition. Research that is cast in terms of these very limited, narrow-band models and, even more so, research that is essentially atheoretical in nature is virtually certain to yield a less-than-comprehensive explanation of learning disabilities.

As an example of an alternative to this conceptually limited approach, a componential analysis of academic and other types of learning should sensitize the researcher to the possibility that, whereas some subtypes of learning-disabled children may experience learning problems because of deficiencies in certain perceptual, cognitive, or behavioral skills, others may manifest such problems as a more direct result of attitudinal or motivational problems or of vastly different perceptual, cognitive, or behavioral difficulties. It should also be clear that different patterns of perceptual, cognitive, and behavioral skills and abilities may encourage different types or degrees of learning difficulties. Recently, theories that emphasize this type of comprehensive, componential approach to the design of developmental neuropsychological explanatory models in this area have emerged (e.g., Fletcher & Taylor, 1984). Our own efforts in this regard (Rourke, 1982, 1987, 1988b) are described in subsequent chapters of this book.

2. Definition of Learning Disabilities. There has been no consistent formulation of the criteria for identifying learning disabilities in the contrasting-groups genre of study. For example, most studies of this ilk employ vaguely defined or even undefined groups, and others use the ratings of teachers and other school personnel, which remain otherwise specified. Some even employ the guidelines of a particular political jurisdiction to define learning disabilities! It is obvious that this lack of clarity and consistency has had a negative impact on the generalizability of even the limited findings of such studies.

Clear, consensually validatable definitions are an urgent need in this area of investigation. In this connection, it would seem patently obvious that the very definitions themselves should be a *result* of sophisticated subtype analysis rather than the starting point of such inquiry (Morris & Fletcher, 1988; Rourke, 1983a, 1983b, 1985; Rourke & Gates, 1981).

3. Developmental Considerations. Part and parcel of the contrasting-groups approach to the study of learning-disabled youngsters is a gross insensitivity to age differences and developmental considerations. Several studies offer support for the notion that the nature and patterning of the skill and ability deficits of some subtypes of learning-disabled children vary with age (e.g., Fisk & Rourke, 1979; Fletcher & Satz, 1980; McKinney, Short, & Feagans, 1985; Morris, Blashfield, & Satz, 1986; Ozols & Rourke, 1988; Rourke, Dietrich, & Young, 1973). Since it would seem reasonable to infer that the neuropsychological functioning of some subtypes of learning-disabled children varies as a function of age (considered as one index of developmental change), the aforementioned inconsistencies in contrasting-groups research results could reflect differences in the ages of the subjects employed.

Although this possibility is sometimes acknowledged by investigators who employ this type of methodology, such a realization has, until quite recently, been the exception rather than the rule. Be that as it may, it is abundantly clear that more cross-sectional and longitudinal studies are necessary in order to clarify the nature of those developmental changes that appear to take place in some learning-disabled children. It is also clear that attention to the issues involved in the study of developmental changes in learning-disabled children is an almost direct function of the sophistication in subtype analysis exhibited by the neuropsychological investigators in this area. (See Morris et al., 1986, for an especially good example of sensitivity to such issues.) Unfortunately, those who pay little or no attention to subtype analysis also demonstrate little or no regard for the developmental changes in these children.

4. Treatment Considerations. Practical experience with children who exhibit marked learning disabilities clearly shows that only some of these individuals respond positively to particular forms of treatment. It is also the case that some forms of treatment for some learning-disabled children are actually counterproductive (Rourke, 1980). Once again, subtype analysis can help to clarify a situation created by the application of the results of contrasting-groups methodology. For example, Lyon (1985) has demonstrated that specific subtypes of disabled readers respond very differently to synthetic phonics and "sight-word" approaches to reading instruction. Sweeney and Rourke (1985) also demonstrated what appeared to be an overreliance of phonetically accurate disabled spellers on the phonetic analysis of individual words, to the apparent detriment of their reading speed.

Idiographic or Idiosyncratic Approach

A strictly individualistic standpoint in this field, although attractive from some clinical perspectives, is viable on neither practical (applied/clinical) nor theoretical grounds. It is patently obvious that persons with learning disabilities are unique. It is also the case that most of them can be classified into homogeneous subtypes on the basis of sets of shared relative strengths and deficiencies in neuropsychological skills and abilities. That is, they have enough in common to be grouped (i.e., subtyped) for the purpose of some important aspects of treatment as well as for specific model-testing purposes. The fact that models based upon subtype analysis can, in fact, be shown to be internally consistent and externally (including ecologically) valid suggests strongly that one need not adopt a position that maintains that each and every individual learning-disabled child is so implacably unique that nothing can be said about his/her development and prognosis and the preferred mode of intervention or treatment. That treatment effects such as those demonstrated by Lyon (1985) obtain is also sufficient proof that strict individualism is not necessary.

In order to accomplish the very desirable goals of scientific and clinical generalizability while insuring the individual applicability of the "general" results of studies in this area, it is necessary to be able to demonstrate that each individual who falls within a particular learning-disability subtype exhibits a very close approximation to the pattern of neuropsychological abilities and deficits that characterizes the subtype as a whole. This should "satisfy" the individualistic criterion while main-

taining the generalizability of treatment and hypothesis-testing imperatives of scientific investigations within this area. The possibility of obtaining this degree of individuation of group results will be particularly
apparent in subsequent chapters of this book, where we will examine
such issues in relationship to the NLD syndrome.

Learning Disabilities as a Heterogeneous Group of Disorders (Subtypes)

Scientific investigation of learning disability subtypes emerged primarily
from careful clinical observations of children who were assessed because
they were thought to be experiencing perceptual and/or learning disabilities. Astute observers, such as Johnson and Myklebust (1967), noted very
clear differences in the patterns of abilities and deficits exhibited by such
children and that specific variations in developmental problems (e.g.,
learning to read) appeared to stem from these differences. In other words,
equally impaired *levels* of learning appeared to result from quite different
etiologies, as suggested in patterns of relative perceptual and cognitive
strengths and weaknesses.

The search for subtypes of learning disabilities took on added importance when it was inferred that these potentially isolatable patterns of
perceptual and cognitive strengths and weaknesses, which were thought to
be responsible for learning difficulties, might be more or less amenable to
different modes of intervention. Indeed, the "subtype by treatment interaction" hypothesis—that is, the notion that the tailoring of specific forms of
treatment to the underlying abilities and deficits of learning-disabled children would be advantageous—was alive and well very early in the history
of the field (e.g., Kirk & McCarthy, 1961). This constituted a second
clinical issue that encouraged researchers to seek a determination of subtype differences among such children. Indeed, many researchers and professionals in the field virtually *assumed* that the matching of the intervention
to the underlying strengths and weaknesses of the child would be the most
efficient and effective therapeutic course to follow.

Positions of this sort were mirrored in the studies conducted by
Johnson and Myklebust (1967) and later by Mattis, French, and Rapin
(1975). These investigators employed an essentially clinical approach to
the identification of subtypes. This rather important thrust to research
was accompanied in the late 1970s by that of investigators who sought to
isolate reliable subtypes of learning-disabled children through the use of

statistical algorithms such as *Q*-type factor analysis and cluster analysis (e.g., Doehring & Hoshko, 1977; Doehring, Hoshko, & Bryans, 1979; Fisk & Rourke, 1979; Petrauskas & Rourke, 1979).

Some of the work in this area is discussed in Chapter 2. At this point, it is sufficient to point out that the use of statistical algorithms to assist in the generating of reliable subtypes of learning disabilities is well under way in this decade (e.g., Joschko & Rourke, 1985; Morris, Blashfield, & Satz, 1981). There are clear indications that this type of systematic search for reliable subtypes of learning-disabled children has begun to have a profoundly positive effect on investigative efforts in this area (Rourke, 1985). Furthermore, systematic attempts at establishing the concurrent, predictive, and construct validity of such subtypes have been proceeding apace (e.g., Fletcher, 1985; Lyon, 1985).

Examples of some of the research carried out in our laboratory that has been designed to grapple with the set of difficulties and imperatives just outlined are discussed in the next chapter. Before presenting these results, however, it is necessary to place this program of research within the context of a general approach to the neuropsychological investigation of central processing abilities and deficits in both learning-disabled and frankly brain-damaged youngsters. (The heuristic advantages of the "marriage" of these two sets of research programs will become more apparent as the book unfolds.)

A SYSTEMATIC DEVELOPMENTAL NEUROPSYCHOLOGICAL APPROACH TO THE STUDY OF LEARNING DISABILITIES

A developmental neuropsychological approach to the study of learning disabilities seeks to understand problems in learning by studying developmental change in behavior as seen through the perspective of brain–behavior models. It is thus an approach that combines the study of development of the brain with the study of the development of behavior. It involves research strategies that pay as much attention to the development of an individual's approach to material to be learned as they do to the accompanying electrophysiological correlates at the level of the cerebral hemispheres. In other words, it is a systematic attempt to fashion a complete understanding of brain–behavior relationships as these are mirrored in the development of central processing abilities and deficits throughout the life-span.

It is unfortunate that the use of a neuropsychological framework such as this for the investigation of learning disabilities in children has so often been misinterpreted as reflecting an emphasis on static, intractable (and therefore limited) notions of the effects of brain impairment on behavior. Indeed, although specific statements to the contrary have been made on many occasions (e.g., Rourke, 1975, 1978b), many otherwise competent researchers and clinicians persist in the notion that such an approach *assumes* that brain damage, disorder, or dysfunction lies at the basis of learning disabilities. Nothing could be further from the truth, since the thrust of much work in this area (see Benton, 1975; Rourke, 1975, 1978a; Taylor & Fletcher, 1983) has been to *demonstrate* whether and to what extent such might be the case.

Be that as it may, the emphasis that my colleagues and I have brought to this enterprise is one that attempts to integrate dimensions of individual and social development on the one hand with relevant central processing features on the other, in order to fashion a useful model with which to study crucial aspects of perception, cognition, and other dimensions of human development. That models and explanatory concepts developed with this aim in mind (e.g., Rourke, 1976b, 1982, 1983b, 1987) contain explanations that are thought to apply both to some types of frankly brain-damaged and learning-disabled children as well as to some aspects of normal human development should come as no surprise, since maximum generalizability is one goal of any scientific model or theory. Specifically with respect to the learning-disabled child, the aspects of these concepts and models that are most relevant are those that have to do with proposed linkages between patterns of central processing abilities and deficits that may predispose a youngster to predictably different patterns of social as well as academic learning disabilities. In addition, these models are designed to encompass developmental change and outcome in patterns of learning and behavioral responsivity.

In the neuropsychology of learning disabilities, the important relationships to bear in mind are those that obtain between *patterns* of performance and *models* of developmental brain–behavior relationships. This is not meant to imply something as trite as the idea that learning disabilities are the *result* of brain damage or dysfunction. Indeed, even were such a cause–effect relationship shown to be the case, it would carry few if any corollaries for the understanding of developmental brain–behavior relationships or for their treatment.

This is also not to suggest that brain–behavior relationships are of little or no importance in the study of learning disabilities. Far from it!

Rather, it is simply the case that we currently understand much more about the psychological than about the neurological aspects of neuropsychological interactions. In other words, we are at much the same stage of theorizing about the latter interactions as was Donald Hebb at the time he composed his landmark monograph, *Organization of Behavior* (1949). Far from discouraging us from pursuing research and model building in this area, the seminal heuristic influence of Hebb's work in general neuropsychology should serve to remind us that the patterns of interaction among brain, development, and behavior, though sometimes exquisitely hypothesized, are still largely unexplored and must be the subject of rigorous scientific testing (Taylor, 1983). For these and other reasons, we chose to study developmental patterns of neuropsychological abilities and deficits within a context provided by the results of neuropsychological research relating to subtypes of learning-disabled children. This effort transpired simultaneously with attempts to understand these important neurodevelopmental relationships in children with demonstrable brain damage. Important upshots of our efforts in this area to date have been the isolating of the NLD syndrome and the formulation of the NLD model.

With the foregoing as background, we examine first the historical roots of the NLD syndrome.[1]

---

[1]At this point, it might be well for the reader to skip ahead to pp. 80–88 in Chapter 5 for a brief look at the elements (i.e., assets and deficits) that constitute the NLD syndrome (Table 5.1) and the dynamics of the syndrome (Figure 5.1). This review might aid in the understanding of the material contained in Chapters 2, 3, and 4 that precedes these formulations.

CHAPTER TWO

Learning Disability Subtype Studies

The identification of the NLD syndrome emerged from our systematic study of learning disability subtypes. The syndrome was not apparent, as such, early on in our investigative efforts. Rather, it took on form and new dimensions as a series of interrelated studies unfolded. Since they were instrumental in defining the NLD syndrome and in formulating the current NLD working model, it would be well to review these studies briefly before discussing the syndrome and the model in detail. Throughout this chapter, an attempt is made to highlight the genesis of this theoretical formulation and to suggest the impact that an investigative tack such as the one described herein may have on the neuropsychology of learning disabilities and on the scientific and applied aspects of child clinical neuropsychology.

Note on Format. Comments on research methodology are interspersed throughout this chapter. These comments are set in italics so as to alert the reader to the momentary interruption in the flow of the chapter that they constitute. This format was felt to be preferable to the insertion of footnotes for this purpose.

CRITERIA FOR DESIGNATION OF CHILDREN AS LEARNING DISABLED

It is important to note that, except where specifically stated to the contrary, the subjects employed in the series of investigations to be reviewed in this chapter met fairly standard criteria for inclusion in studies of learning-disabled youngsters (Rourke, 1975, 1976b, 1978b).

That is, these children

1. Were markedly deficient in at least one school subject area.
2. Obtained Wechsler Intelligence Scale for Children (WISC) Full Scale IQs within the roughly normal range.
3. Were free of primary emotional disturbance.
4. Had adequate visual and auditory acuity.
5. Lived in homes and communities where socioeconomic deprivation was not a factor.
6. Had experienced only the usual childhood illnesses.
7. Had attended school regularly since the age of 5½ or 6 years.

In addition, all subjects spoke English as their native language.

The importance of an appreciation of these criteria for what we may term a "general" definition of children with learning disabilities will become more apparent as we proceed to both more generic and more specific definitions of this heterogeneous entity (see especially Chapter 8). For now, it is sufficient to note that the generalizability of the results of the studies to be discussed in this chapter must be viewed within the context of the general "exclusionary" criteria that were employed in the selection of subjects for them.

WISC VERBAL IQ–PERFORMANCE IQ DISCREPANCIES

Study 1

The first study in the series (Rourke, Young, & Flewelling, 1971) involved learning-disabled children who were chosen on the basis of Verbal Intelligence Quotient (VIQ) and Performance Intelligence Quotient (PIQ) discrepancies on the Wechsler Intelligence Scale for Children (WISC; Wechsler, 1949). The study was designed to assess the relationships between such discrepancies and selected verbal, auditory-perceptual, visual-perceptual, and problem-solving abilities. Three groups, each containing 30 learning-disabled children, were formed on the basis of the relationship between their VIQ and PIQ scores on the WISC: one group, designated HP–LV (for high performance and low verbal scores), consisted of subjects whose PIQ scores were at least 10 points higher than their VIQs. A second group, labeled V = P, was composed of subjects with VIQ and PIQ within 4 points of each other. The third group, designated HV–LP, had VIQ values at least 10 points higher than their PIQ. All subjects fell within a Full Scale WISC range of 79 to 119 and an age range of 9 to 14 years; there were no significant differences in either WISC Full Scale IQ or age among the three groups.

As expected, the performance of the HV–LP group was superior to that of the HP–LV group on those tasks that involved verbal and auditory-perceptual skills, including the Peabody Picture Vocabulary Test (PPVT; Dunn, 1965); Aphasia Screening, Speech-Sounds Perception, and Seashore Rhythm Tests (Reitan & Davison, 1974); and the Reading, Spelling and Arithmetic subtests of the Wide Range Achievement Test (WRAT; Jastak & Jastak, 1965). The differences on all but the PPVT were statistically significant. The performances of the HP–LV group were, as expected, superior to those of the HV–LP group on tasks that primarily involved visual-perceptual skills, including the Trail Making Test (TMT), Part A, and Target Test (Reitan & Davison, 1974). Also as expected, the performance of the V=P group occupied positions roughly intermediate between those of the other two groups over most of the dependent measures. Although the difference was not statistically significant, the HP–LV group did somewhat better than did the HV–LP group on the Category Test (Reitan & Davison, 1974).

Of particular importance in the present context were two additional findings of this study that had not been anticipated. First, the HV–LP group did well on the TMT, Part B, relative to Part A, whereas the HP–LV group did poorly on TMT, Part B, relative to Part A. This was thought to be the case because the HV–LP group, although relatively deficient in the visual-perceptual abilities necessary for success on both parts of the TMT, were relatively more adept than the HP–LV group at the verbal and symbolic abilities necessary for success on TMT, Part B.

Second, an *a posteriori* comparison of the Reading, Spelling, and Arithmetic subtests of the WRAT within each of the three groups indicated a striking, statistically significant difference between Reading and Spelling (high) on the one hand and Arithmetic (low) on the other hand for the HV–LP group. Although no such statistically significant differences in performance on these three subtests of the WRAT were present in either of the other two groups, there was an opposite trend evident in the performance of the HP–LV group, that is, a tendency toward higher performance on the WRAT Arithmetic subtest relative to performance on the WRAT Reading and Spelling subtests.

One important implication of the results of this investigation is that, for older (9- to 14-year-old) children, the WISC VIQ–PIQ relationship appears to be a far more important consideration with regard to learning disabilities than is general level of psychometric intelligence. That is, although the three groups of learning-disabled children were equated for WISC Full Scale IQ, their vastly different patterns of relative cognitive strengths and weaknesses became evident when a more complex type of IQ characterization was employed, namely, VIQ–PIQ discrepancies. Indeed, although we did not emphasize this point at the time, it appeared that the groups we had formed on the basis of WISC VIQ–PIQ discrepancies might very well constitute unique subtypes within the learning-disabled population. This appeared to be so not only for independent measures of verbal, auditory-perceptual, and visual-spatial abilities, but also for patterns of performance on the Reading, Spelling, and Arithmetic subtests of the WRAT. Subsequent examinations of all these dimensions have demonstrated that, in large measure, this seems to be the case (see Fletcher, 1985).

A further note regarding these findings is that the pattern of relative abilities (verbal and auditory-perceptual) and deficits (visual-spatial) exhibited by the HV–LP group is similar to what would be expected in adults who are experiencing the debilitating effects of a significant lesion confined to the right cerebral hemisphere. Furthermore, the opposite pattern of relative abilities and deficits exhibited by the HP–LV group is similar to what would be expected in adults experiencing a similar left-hemisphere lesion. Since these groups of learning-disabled children with different configurations of VIQ–PIQ discrepancies exhibited patterns of performance that might suggest differential impairment of skills ordinarily thought to be subserved primarily by one or the other of the two cerebral hemispheres, it was thought advisable to carry out a subsequent investigation including dependent variables from a very different adaptive domain, so as to shed some additional light on this interesting theoretical question.

Study 2

For this second study, three groups of subjects who exhibited patterns of VIQ–PIQ discrepancies virtually identical to those in the Rourke, Young, and Flewelling (1971) investigation were selected, in order to compare their performances on motor and psychomotor tasks that allowed for separate assessments of right-hand and left-hand efficiency (Rourke & Telegdy, 1971). The motor and psychomotor tasks used were chosen to represent varying degrees of two dimensions: (1) complexity and (2) the visual-spatial skills necessary for success. Thus, the dependent measures ranged from relatively simple motor tasks (e.g., strength of grip, speed of tapping) to relatively complex psychomotor tasks (e.g., timed placement of grooved pegs into holes).The 45 male learning-disabled children (15 each in the HP–LV, V=P and HV–LP groups) selected for study were between the ages of 9 and 14 years, and their WISC Full Scale IQs fell within the range of 85 to 115. There were no statistically significant differences between the groups in terms of age or WISC Full Scale IQ.

The performance of these three groups of subjects on 25 measures indicated clear superiority of the HP–LV group (especially in comparison to the HV–LP group) on most measures of complex motor and psychomotor abilities, regardless of the hand employed. The clearest separation of the groups was observed on the most complex psychomotor measure employed (Grooved Pegboard Test; Klove, 1963). On this task, the differences were evident for both right- and left-hand trials, with the following pattern of relative superiority between groups obtaining: HP–LV > V=P > HV–LP. There were nonsignificant trends in evidence favoring the right-hand over the left-hand performances of the HV–LP group on the Finger Tapping (Reitan & Davison, 1974) and Tactual Performance Tests (Reitan & Davison, 1974), with the opposite pattern of right-hand and left-hand results for the HP–LV group. These findings, in addition to the superior performance of the HP–LV over the HV–LP group on the Location component of the Tactual Performance Test, offered support for one of the alternative hypotheses of the study, that is, that the HP–LV group, because of relative superiority in visual-perceptual skills, would do better than the HV–LP group on tasks involving complex visual-motor coordination and spatial visualization and memory. Although expectations involving differential hand superiority of the HP–LV and HV–LP groups were not supported, the results were considered consistent with the view that WISC VIQ–PIQ discrepancies reflect the differential integrity of the two cerebral hemispheres in older children with learning disabilities.

Conclusions: Studies 1 and 2

The important conclusions and hypotheses formulated at this point in our research program were as follows.

1. It was apparent that older (9- to 14-year-old) learning-disabled children did not constitute a homogeneous group. There were clearly significant differences between the patterns of abilities and deficits exhibited by our three groups of learning disabled youngsters. However, there was still a need to determine the reliability of these apparent subtypes.

2. Simply separating these learning-disabled children for study on the basis of WISC VIQ–PIQ discrepancies suggested strongly that one subtype within this group (HV–LP) seemed to be relatively efficient in skills and abilities ordinarily thought to be subserved primarily by the left cerebral hemisphere (e.g., speech-sounds discrimination), whereas another subtype (HP–LV) appeared to be much more efficient in skills and abilities ordinarily thought to be subserved primarily by the right cerebral hemisphere (e.g., visual-spatial-organizational skills). (This hypothesis was to be subjected to several different tests throughout the course of this research program.)

3. The consequences of the separation of the groups in terms of WISC VIQ–PIQ discrepancies vis-à-vis differences in levels and patterns of performance in reading, spelling, and arithmetic appeared to be important. At this point, it seemed reasonable to investigate the possible neuropsychological significance of such patterns of academic achievement.

Before pursuing these implications further, however, we felt it necessary to investigate the correlates of VIQ–PIQ discrepancies among younger children with learning disabilities, in the hope of revealing some developmental implications regarding their emerging abilities and deficits. Although the patterns of abilities and deficits exhibited by the 9- to 14-year-olds studied to this point appeared to be interpretable in terms of fairly well-established principles of brain–behavior relationships that had been generated in the study of adults, we were not so sanguine as to assume that such would be the case for children at more tender ages. Indeed, there appeared to be rather sound reasons for thinking otherwise, including those of a psychometric (higher variability in performance on the versions of the tests used at younger ages) and a developmental (less "differentiation" of abilities at younger ages) nature.

Study 3

In the third study of this series (Rourke, Dietrich, & Young, 1973), 82 learning-disabled children aged 5 to 8 years were divided into three groups, using virtually the same criteria as those employed in the Rourke, Young, and Flewelling (1971) and Rourke and Telegdy (1971) investigations. The children had WISC Full Scale IQs ranging from 79 to 120; there were no significant differences between the groups with respect to age and Full Scale IQ. The study employed as dependent variables several measures within the following two categories: (1) verbal, auditory-perceptual, visual-perceptual, and problem-solving tests similar to those employed in the Rourke et al. (1971) study; and (2) motor and psychomotor tests similar to those employed by Rourke and Telegdy (1971).

In contrast to the findings of Rourke et al. (1971) and Rourke and Telegdy (1971), there were few significant differences in performance evident among the three groups in this third study. However, the pattern of group differences on the PPVT, WRAT, Speech-Sounds Perception Test, Seashore Rhythm Test, Category Test, and Target Test closely resembled that exhibited by the 9- to 14-year-old children in the Rourke et al. (1971) study. The only statistically significant differences evident among the motor and psychomotor measures indicated superiority of the HP–LV group over the HV–LP group on selected aspects of the Mazes (Klove, 1963), Grooved Pegboard, and Tactual Performance Tests. Given the large number of comparisons carried out, the latter differences may have emerged by chance.

Although the pattern of performance on the verbal, auditory-perceptual, and visual-perceptual measures exhibited by these 5- to 8-year-old subjects was of interest because of its similarity to results obtained with older learning-disabled children, the absence of any strong indications of differences in motor and psychomotor patterns and the relatively large variability of performances across the majority of measures at this age level suggested strongly that meaningful developmental patterns would be difficult to determine with these data. One thing was abundantly clear, however: There was an emerging differentiation of abilities in learning-disabled children similar to that seen with great regularity in normal children. In addition, this progressive differentiation of abilities appeared to be accompanied by an emerging differentiation of selective deficits in these subtypes of learning-disabled youngsters.

Conclusions: Developmental Dimensions

At this juncture, it would be well to mention three important developmental dimensions relating to the abilities and deficits of learning-disabled children, which were evident in the cross-sectional comparisons afforded by the first three studies:

1. The notion that some skills and abilities crucial for various types of learning can lag behind and then "catch up," whereas others are deficient and tend to stay that way over time, has been the subject of

much inquiry in developmental neuropsychology (e.g., Rourke, 1976c; Usprich, 1976). These are important considerations with respect to these studies, but it would be well to hold off discussing them in depth until the results of other investigations that bear on this topic are presented.

2. Another concept that may be important for our understanding of the emerging deficits is "psychic edema" (Rourke, 1983b). This concept was arrived at by analogy with the general effects (edema) of significant craniocerebral trauma and the gradually emerging prominence of specific adaptive deficits as these more general effects subside. The notion of psychic edema suggests that attentional deficit and other more general effects of disordered neural development may subside with advancing years, with a correlative emergence of deficits in information processing that have been extant from the child's earliest years but which were effectively masked by these more general disturbances. This notion will arise in subsequent discussions of what constitutes change in information processing capacities over time, as well as which factors mitigate against being able to measure such changes in a reliable and valid fashion.

3. One final developmental implication of the results of the series of studies reviewed to this point should be mentioned. It appeared to us that further investigation of hypotheses relating to the differential integrity of left- and right-hemisphere systems as these relate to patterns of abilities and deficits in various subtypes of learning-disabled children would best be accomplished by in-depth study of the 9- to 14-year-old group. An example of this is the set of studies, discussed below, that focused on specific patterns of WRAT Reading, Spelling, and Arithmetic performances within this age group.

General Conclusions of Studies 1, 2, and 3

The studies reviewed to this point would also suggest that the following *general* conclusions are tenable:

1. There are subtypes of children with learning disabilities that can be identified and studied in a reliable fashion.

2. Some distinct patterns of "cognitive" abilities and deficits are associated with equally distinct patterns of sensorimotor abilities and deficits in different subtypes of learning-disabled children. These are especially evident among older (9- to 14-year-old) learning-disabled children.

3. There are significant developmental differences in the manifestations of learning disabilities and in the associations between and among

these manifestations. Specifically, manifestations of learning disabilities in 9- to 14-year-children are rather consistent with expectations based upon models of brain–behavior relationships derived from studies of normal and brain-damaged adults; such manifestations in 5- to 8-year-old children, for the most part, are not in line with these expectations.

PATTERNS OF READING, SPELLING, AND ARITHMETIC

We turn now to a review of those studies that were designed to determine the neuropsychological significance of patterns of academic achievement. As mentioned earlier, these investigations were stimulated by the unexpected patterns of WRAT Reading, Spelling, and Arithmetic performances that turned up in the VIQ–PIQ discrepancy studies. Specifically, we were interested in determining whether children who exhibit particular patterns of WRAT Reading, Spelling, and Arithmetic performances would also exhibit predictable patterns of neuropsychological abilities and deficits.

Study 4

In the first of these investigations (Rourke & Finlayson, 1978), learning-disabled children between the ages of 9 and 14 years were divided into three groups (15 subjects in each group) on the basis of their patterns of performance in reading and spelling tasks relative to their level of performance in arithmetic. The three groups were equated for age and WISC Full Scale IQ. The subjects in group 1 were uniformly deficient in reading, spelling, and arithmetic. Group 2 was composed of subjects whose arithmetic performance, although clearly below age expectation, was significantly better than their performance in reading and spelling. The subjects in group 3 exhibited normal reading and spelling and markedly impaired arithmetic performance. Although *all three groups performed well below age expectation in arithmetic*, the performance of groups 2 and 3 was superior to that of group 1; *groups 2 and 3 did not differ from one another in their impaired levels of arithmetic performance.*

Note on Research Methodology. It is clear that, in the traditional contrasting-groups type of study of arithmetic disability, children from groups 1, 2, and 3 would have "qualified" for admission to the "disabled arithmetic" group. The alarming shortcomings of such a research design are well illustrated by the results of the studies under consideration.

The three groups' performance on 16 dependent measures, chosen in the light of the results of previous studies in this series (particularly study 1, Rourke, Young, & Flewelling, 1971), were compared. The results of this investigation may be summarized as follows: (1) the performance of groups 1 and 2 was superior to that of group 3 on measures of visual-perceptual and visual-spatial abilities (e.g., WISC Block Design, Target Test), and (2) group 3 performed at superior levels to groups 1 and 2 on measures of verbal and auditory-perceptual abilities (e.g., WISC Vocabulary, Speech-Sounds Perception Test). In the context of the results of the previous studies in this series, it was notable that all subjects in group 1 had a lower VIQ than PIQ, that 14 of the 15 subjects in group 2 had a lower VIQ than PIQ (one subject had equivalent VIQ and PIQ), and that all subjects in group 3 had a higher VIQ than PIQ.

It is clear that groups 1 and 2 performed in a fashion very similar to that expected of groups of older children with learning disabilities who exhibit the WISC HP–LV pattern, and that group 3 performed in a manner expected of older children with learning disabilities who exhibit the WISC HV–LP pattern (Rourke, Young, & Flewelling, 1971). It is also important to emphasize that *individual subjects* within the three groups exhibited results on the WISC that were all but indistinguishable from the *group* results just reported. Thus, this type of nomothetic research tack did not do violence to any idiosyncratic (idiographic) imperatives, at least in terms of WISC VIQ–PIQ discrepancies.

If there is a reason to believe that WISC VIQ–PIQ discrepancies may be associated with or reflect the differential integrity of the two cerebral hemispheres in older children with learning disabilities, as has already been suggested, then it would appear that the basis on which the groups were chosen in this fourth study may also reflect this difference. At the very least, the results would be consistent with the view that the subjects in group 3 may be limited in their performance because of compromised functional integrity of the right cerebral hemisphere, and that the subjects in groups 1 and 2 were suffering from the adverse effects of relatively dysfunctional left-hemisphere systems. These inferences were felt to be reasonable because the subjects in group 3 did particularly poorly *only* in those skills and abilities ordinarily thought to be subserved primarily by the right cerebral hemisphere, whereas the subjects in groups 1 and 2 were markedly deficient *only* in those skills and abilities ordinarily thought to be subserved primarily by the left cerebral hemisphere.

Also of importance in the present context was the fact that the two groups of subjects who had been equated for deficient arithmetic performance (groups 2 and 3) exhibited vastly different performance on verbal and visual-spatial tasks. These differences were clearly related to their *patterns* of reading, spelling, and arithmetic rather than to their *levels of performance* in arithmetic per se. Indeed, although the WRAT Reading, Spelling, and Arithmetic subtest scores of group 2 were in no case significantly superior to those of group 3, the performance of group 2 was significantly superior to that of group 3 on all of the measures of visual-perceptual and visual-spatial skills employed in this investigation (WISC Picture Completion, Picture Arrangement, Block Design, and Object Assembly; Target Test). More generally, it seemed reasonable to infer that the neuropsychological bases for the impaired arithmetic performance of groups 2 and 3 differed markedly: Whereas subjects in the group 2 subtype would appear to experience difficulty in mechanical arithmetic because of "verbal" deficiencies, subjects of the group 3 subtype would be expected to encounter similar difficulties as a direct result of deficiencies in visual-spatial abilities. Indeed, a qualitative analysis of the errors made by these two subtypes of learning-disabled youngsters, which will be discussed later, suggests very strongly that this is, in fact, the case.

Note on Research Methodology. The methodological implications of such findings for research in children's learning disabilities is quite clear: Were subjects from groups 2 and 3 combined to form a single group defined as "disabled in arithmetic" for the purpose of parametric investigation, comparisons of measures of central tendency between such a combined group and a group performing at a normal level in arithmetic would severely distort and mask the very marked differences in verbal and visual-spatial abilities exhibited by these two learning disability subtypes. In addition, it would appear to be the case that children of these subtypes require different modes of educational intervention in order to make academic progress in their areas of deficiency (Rourke, Bakker, Fisk, & Strang, 1983; Rourke & Strang, 1983; Strang & Rourke, 1985b) and should be subjected to "educational validation" study (see Lyon, 1985, for an example of this type of investigation).

Study 5

In this study, we decided to determine whether these same three groups of 9- to 14-year-old learning-disabled subjects would differ in predictable ways on tests from a very different neuropsychological domain, namely those designed to measure motor, psychomotor, and tactile-perceptual skills. In this investigation (Rourke & Strang, 1978), we were particularly interested to determine if any evidence might be adduced to support a view that these groups of learning-disabled children were suffering from differential impairment of functional systems thought to be subserved primarily by structures and systems within the left or the right cerebral hemisphere. We hoped to accomplish this through an analysis of the right- and left-hand performance of these groups of right-handed learning-disabled children on selected motor, psychomotor, and tactile-perceptual measures.

The motor tests included the Finger Tapping Test and the Strength of Grip Test (Reitan & Davison, 1974). The psychomotor measures included the time measures for the Maze Test, the Grooved Pegboard Test, and the Tactual Performance Test (Klove, 1963; Reitan & Davison, 1974). The tests for tactile-perceptual disturbances were those described in Reitan and Davison (1974), as follows: Finger Agnosia, Finger-Tip Number-Writing Perception, and Coin Recognition. A summary score that included all errors on the latter tests for tactile-perceptual disturbances for each hand was derived for use in the study. The principal results of this investigation and their implications for the current discussion are as follows.

There were no statistically significant differences between or among the groups on the simple motor measures, over and above those that would be expected to be exhibited by the exlusively right-handed children employed in this study. The expected superiority of performance for groups 1 and 2 over that of group 3 was clearly in evidence on two of the complex psychomotor measures (Maze and Grooved Pegboard Tests). Differential hand superiority was found between the groups only on the Tactual Performance Test. Groups 1 and 3 displayed a pattern of poor left-hand performance relative to right-hand performance on this measure, whereas the exact opposite was true for group 2. The left-hand performance of group 2 was significantly superior to that of groups 1 and 3. In line with the patterns evident for the Maze and Grooved Pegboard Tests, the performance of groups 1 and 2 on the "both hands" measure of the Tactual Performance Test was superior to that of group 3. Finally, comparisons favoring the performance of groups 1 and 2 over that of group 3 on the composite tactile-perceptual measure were significant for both the right and left hands. There was also a tendency evident among subjects in group 3 for their right-hand performance to be superior to that with the left hand.

Thus it was demonstrated that learning-disabled children in group 3 have marked deficiencies relative to groups 1 and 2 in some psychomotor and tactile-perceptual skills. In addition, comparisons of these results with the norms available for these tests (Knights & Norwood, 1980) indicated that the performance of group 3 fell well below age-expectation on these measures, whereas the performance of groups 1 and 2 was well within normal limits.

The very marked discrepancy between the performance of groups 2 and 3 on the Tactual Performance Test would offer clear support for the hypothesis regarding differential hemispheric integrity for these two groups, which was advanced in connection with study 4 (Rourke & Finlayson, 1978). Confining our discussion to the performance of groups 2 and 3 in the two studies under consideration, it is clear that group 2 scored lower than expected on measures of abilities ordinarily thought to be subserved primarily by systems within the left cerebral hemisphere, and much better (in an age-appropriate fashion) on measures of abilities ordinarily thought to be subserved primarily by right-hemisphere systems. The opposite state of affairs obtained for children of the group 3 subtype.

Conclusions: Studies 4 and 5

A comparison of the results of this fifth study with those of study 4 is especially important in the case of group 3. The particular pattern that emerged for this group is one that is somewhat analogous to that seen in the Gerstmann syndrome (Benson & Geschwind, 1970; Kinsbourne & Warrington, 1963). That is, the children in group 3 exhibited the following: outstanding deficiencies in arithmetic (within a context of normal reading and spelling); visual-spatial orientation difficulties, including right–left orientation problems; general psychomotor incoordination, including problems that would fall under the rubric of "dysgraphia"; and impaired tactile-discrimination abilities, including finger agnosia. At the same time, it must be emphasized that the patterning of abilities and deficits exhibited by children in group 3 would appear to be most compatible with relatively deficient *right*-hemisphere systems, rather than with deficient *left*-hemisphere systems, as advanced by Benson and Geschwind (1970).

The results of the Rourke and Finlayson (1978) and the Rourke and Strang (1978) investigations would appear to have significant and widespread import for the academic and social remediation of such children (see Strang & Rourke, 1985a; also see Chapters 3 and 7) and for the determination of subtypes of learning-disabled youngsters (Fletcher, 1985; Rourke, 1983b; Rourke & Strang, 1983; Strang & Rourke, 1985b). Rather than deal with these implications at this juncture, however, it would be instructive to consider the results of the last three studies in this series—one dealing with the concept-formation and problem-solving abilities of 9- to 14-year-old group 2 and 3 children (Strang & Rourke, 1983), and two others dealing with the determination of the verbal, visual–spatial, psychomotor, and tactile-perceptual capacities of 7- to 8-year-old group 1, 2, and 3 children (Ozols & Rourke, 1988, in press).

Before proceeding to a discussion of the next investigation in this series, it would be well to point out the reasons for excluding group 1 from an in-depth analysis in conjunction with this and other studies. Reasons for this relate to the specific aims of this work (i.e., to describe and explain in detail the NLD syndrome and the model designed to encompass and explain its complex manifestations) and to the fact that group 1 appears to be made up of several discrete subtypes of learning-disabled children (Fisk & Rourke, 1979; Petrauskas & Rourke, 1979). Some information regarding the findings of our subtyping studies of "across-the-board" learning disabilities is contained in a subsequent section of this chapter.

Study 6

In this investigation (Strang & Rourke, 1983), 9- to 14-year-old group 2 and 3 children (15 in each group) were chosen in a fashion virtually identical to that employed in studies 4 and 5; that is, the primary criteria for group selection were subjects' patterns of academic performance in reading, spelling, and arithmetic. These groups were equated for age and WISC Full Scale IQ (range: 86–114). The dependent measures employed included the number of errors on the six subtests of the Halstead Category Test (Reitan & Davison, 1974) and the total number of errors scored on the entire test. The form of the Category Test used for children 9 to 15 years of age includes six subtests and 168 items. The sixth subtest includes only review items from subtests 2 through 5 in a randomly ordered fashion. The Category Test is a relatively complex concept-formation measure involving nonverbal abstract reasoning, hypothesis testing, and the ability to benefit from positive and negative informational feedback. The most important results of this study were the following.

As predicted, group 3 children scored significantly higher on the Category Test total errors score than did those in group 2. Furthermore, the level of performance of group 3 children on this measure was approximately one standard deviation below age expectation (Knights & Norwood, 1980), whereas group 2 children performed in an age-appropriate manner. An analysis of performance on the subtests of the Category Test revealed that the performance of group 2 was significantly superior to that of group 3 on the final three subtests (4, 5, and 6). It is notable that subtests 4 and 5 of the Category Test are those that are most complex in terms of their requirements for visual–spatial analysis, and that subtest 6 requires incidental memory for the previously correct solutions. As such, subtest 6 is one measure of the child's capacity to benefit from experience with the task.

These results were expected, in view of the previously documented deficiencies exhibited by group 3 children, which we thought would have interfered with the normal development of the higher-order cognitive skills presumably tapped by the Category Test. Our reasoning was as follows: It would seem highly likely that the majority of children in group 3 have suffered since birth from the ill effects of their neuropsychological deficiencies (i.e., bilateral tactile-perceptual and psychomotor impairment and poorly developed visual-perceptual-organizational abilities). In terms of the theory regarding the development of intellectual functions formulated by Piaget (1954), one would expect that these deficiencies would have a negative effect on the acquisition of cognitive skills at later stages. Piaget's description of what he considered to be significant sensorimotor activities serves to highlight the importance of tactile-perceptual, psychomotor, and visual-perceptual-organizational functions for the infant and young child. Since group 3 children are particularly deficient in these neuropsychological functions (and probably have been so since birth), it would seem highly probable that they have not benefited as much as have most children from the sensorimotor period of development. Furthermore, their cognitive operations, particularly those that are not regulated easily by language functions (e.g., higher-order analysis, organization, and synthesis), would also be expected to be deficient.

The essentially intact Category Test performance of group 2 would suggest strongly that language and thought, as Piaget suggested, are quite distinct. Group 2 youngsters, although deficient in many aspects of linguistic and auditory-perceptual functioning, performed at normal levels on this very complex test of nonverbal concept formation and problem solving. Apart from some difficulties exhibited on subtest 1 (which involves the *reading* of Roman numerals), they performed well within age expectations on the other five subtests. They also exhibited a much better developed capacity to benefit from experience with this task than did the group 3 children. Finally, they showed considerable capacity to deal effectively and adaptively with the novel problem-solving, hypothesis-testing, and cognitive flexibility requirements of the Category Test.

The fact that there is absolutely no evidence of impairment in tactile-perceptual, visual-spatial-organizational, and psychomotor skills in group 2 children would suggest that their course through the sensorimotor period of intellectual development described by Piaget (1954) would have been normal. Even though afflicted with fairly obvious difficulties in the development and elaboration of psycholinguistic skills, their development of higher-order cognitive processes seems to have proceeded without complication. On the other hand, group 3 children exhibit signs of significant impairment in these same skills. It may be the case that these constitute the conceptual underpinnings or "building blocks" for the development of skills involving reasoning (such as mathematics), and that deficiencies in them are responsible for the fact that these children have failed to develop higher-order concept-formation and problem-solving abilities to a normal degree. Whether and to what extent the relative failure in conceptual reasoning and related abilities is a direct function of inadequate sensorimotor experience must wait upon the results of further research.

Summary of Major Findings: Studies 4, 5, and 6

Figure 2.1 is included in order to summarize the major findings of the three studies of 9- to 14-year-old children in groups 2 and 3. Hereafter, these will be referred to as group R-S (Reading and Spelling) and group A

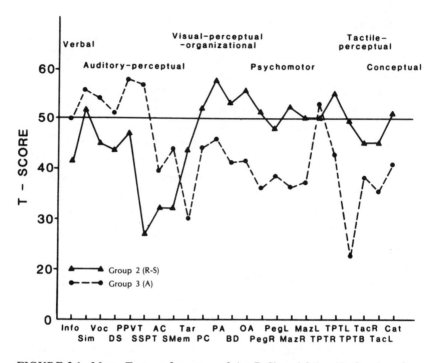

FIGURE 2.1. Mean *T* scores for groups 2 (or R-S) and 3 (or A). Good performance: above 50; poor performance: below 50. Abbreviations: Info, WISC Information; Sim, WISC Similarities; Voc, WISC Vocabulary; DS, WISC Digit Span; PPVT, Peabody Picture Vocabulary Test; SSPT, Speech-Sounds Perception Test; AC, Auditory Closure Test; SMem, Sentence Memory Test; Tar, Target Test; PC, WISC Picture Completion; PA, WISC Picture Arrangement; BD, WISC Block Deisgn; OA, WISC Object Assembly; PegR, Grooved Pegboard Test, right hand; PegL, Grooved Pegboard Test, left hand; MazR, Maze Test, right hand; MazL, Maze Test, left hand; TPTR, Tactual Performance Test, right hand; TPTL, Tactual Performance Test, left hand; TPTB, Tactual Performance Test, both hands; TacR, tactile-perceptual abilities, right hand; TacL, tactile-perceptual abilities, left hand; Cat, Halstead Category Test. From "Arithmetic Disability Subtypes: The Neuropsychological Significance of Specific Arithmetical Impairment in Childhood" by J. D. Strang and B. P. Rourke, in *Neuropsychology of Learning Disabilities: Essentials of Subtype Analysis* edited by B. P. Rourke, New York: Guilford Press, 1985, p. 175. Copyright 1985 by The Guilford Press. Reprinted by permission.

(Arithmetic), respectively; group 1 will be referred to as group R-S-A (Reading, Spelling, and Arithmetic). (See Table 2.1 for a clarification of the designations of these groups in the various studies reviewed to this point.) In Figure 2.1, the T score means are structured in such a way that average performance for the particular age group in question, according to the Knights and Norwood (1980) norms, is represented by $T = 50$, with a standard deviation (SD) of 10. Thus, a T score of 60 represents a level of performance that is one SD above the mean, whereas a T score of 40 represents a score that is one SD below the mean for the particular age group. This use of T scores allows direct comparisons to be made among the various tests in a type of profile analysis; this would not be possible if raw scores were used.

As can be seen in Figure 2.1, the deficiencies, relative to age-based norms, exhibited by group R-S children are virtually confined to the verbal and especially the auditory-perceptual areas. On the other hand, Group A children exhibit deficiencies in a wide variety of visual-perceptual-organizational, psychomotor, tactile-perceptual, and conceptual areas. [Their relative problems with the Auditory Closure Test and the Sentence Memory Test may be a reflection of their difficulties in dealing with novel tasks (Auditory Closure) and their problems in understanding and utilizing semantic content or meaning as a memory aid (Sentence Memory), as would be expected in terms of the Rourke (1982) model (see Chapter 4).]

Qualitative Analysis of Arithmetic Errors

If these generalizations regarding group R-S and group A children are valid in the individual case, one would expect that a qualitative analysis of the mechanical arithmetic performance (or of any other complex performance that is amenable to componential analysis) of individuals from each group would reflect these group differences. Such analyses do, in fact, reflect these differences and their hypothesized neuropsychological roots, as demonstrated by the following.

It should be noted that a child's (or an adult's) errors in arithmetic may vary as a function of such variables as (1) the type of presentation (e.g., written versus oral), (2) other sources of variability that are inherent in the testing situation itself (e.g., time limits), (3) the type and quality of instruction received in mechanical arithmetic, and (4) age or developmental stage. These dimensions need to be borne in mind when considering the quality of errors made by learning-disabled children.

TABLE 2.1. Group Designations Used for Various Studies by Rourke and Colleagues

Rourke, Young, & Flewelling (1971) Rourke & Telegdy (1971) Rourke, Dietrich, & Young (1973)	Rourke & Finlayson (1978) Rourke & Strang (1978) Strang & Rourke (1983)	Rourke (1982) & this book
Group V = P	Group 1	Group R-S-A
Group HP–LV	Group 2	Group R-S
Group HV–LP	Group 3	Group A

Note. There is a rather close comparability between the pairs of designations in the rows of the middle and last columns (i.e., between group 1 and group R-S-A and so on). With regard to the designations in the first and middle columns, group HP–LV is most like groups 1 and 2, and group HV–LP is most like group 3.

When the WRAT arithmetic performances of group R-S children are examined, it is typically found that they make fewer mistakes than is generally the case for children who are deficient in this area. They exhibit a tendency to avoid unfamiliar arithmetic operations or those about which they are uncertain. An exception to this state of affairs is sometimes seen in younger, 9- to 10-year-old children, who seem to find ways to calculate correctly without being entirely familiar with the standard procedures (e.g., they may count on their fingers because they do not remember the multiplication tables). The errors made by these children usually reflect some difficulty in remembering mathematical tables or remembering a particular step in the correct procedure for solving a problem. These children also tend to avoid problems that require the reading of printed words. Virtually all of the problems that group R-S children have with mechanical arithmetic can be summarized in terms of two difficulties: (1) disability in reading and (2) inexperience with the subject material.

With respect to the latter, it should be emphasized that it is typical for older group R-S children to be involved in special educational programs in which reading and spelling activities are emphasized. In such programs, attention to the development of mathematical abilities tends to be rather minimal. In any case, it should be clear that the problems that group R-S children exhibit in the studies described above (i.e., primarily "verbal" in nature) are reflected in a qualitative analysis of their mechanical arithmetic errors. Also reflected is their capacity for understanding when problems are too difficult for them, as well as other forms of adaptive behavior that one would expect to see in children whose nonverbal problem-solving, strategy-generating, hypothesis-testing, and feedback-processing skills are intact.

A qualitative analysis of the mechanical arithmetic errors of group A reveals a far different picture. As was the case for group R-S children, however, the quality of the errors made by group A children is predictable in terms of their pattern of neuropsychological abilities and deficits. The analysis reveals that they tend to make a large number and a wide range of types of errors on the WRAT Arithmetic subtest. As would be expected, the type and, in some cases, the quality of errors varies somewhat with age. Nevertheless, it is found that some of the oldest children in group A persist in making the same types of errors as are found in the WRAT profiles of the younger (9-year-old) children in this group. The most prevalent types of mechanical arithmetic errors that were found in the WRAT Arithmetic profiles of group A children can be classified into seven overlapping categories, as follows:

1. Spatial Organization. Errors in spatial organization include misaligning numbers in columns (e.g., in a two-digit multiplication question) and any problem that a child might experience with directionality (e.g., subtracting the minuend from the subtrahend in a subtraction question).

2. Visual Detail. Misreading the mathematical sign is an example of an error in visual detail, as is failing to include required visual detail in the answer (e.g., a dollar sign or decimal place).

3. Procedural Errors. In some cases, group A children may miss or add a step to a specific mechanical arithmetic procedure; in others, they may apply a learned rule for one mechanical arithmetic procedure to a dissimilar procedure.

4. Failure to Shift Psychological Set. When two or more operations of one kind (e.g., addition) are followed by an operation of another kind (e.g., subtraction), group A children sometimes fail to shift set and, instead, proceed to apply the practiced procedure to the new operation. Other types of procedural errors (see above) can be associated with problems in shifting psychological set as well.

5. Graphomotor Skills. Deficiencies in graphomotor skills include children writing numbers so poorly that they are difficult for them to read, leading to errors in some questions. The tendency of group A children to write with large, rather poorly formed numbers often leads to crowding of work (on the WRAT Arithmetic subtest there is only a fixed amount of space in which to complete each question), which can result in errors. Although graphomotor skills in the case of cursive script (words) tend to become well developed with advancing years, similar advancement in the writing of numbers within calculation procedures is not typical.

6. *Memory.* In some cases, the group A child's errors appear to result from his/her failure to remember a particular number fact, but this type of error is not predominant in the profiles of these children. Often it may be clear that the child has the rule available in memory, but fails to access the remembered rule at the point at which it is needed in the arithmetic calculation process.

7. *Judgment and Reasoning.* Children in this group typically attempt questions that are clearly beyond their current realm of expertise. In these cases, they produce solutions that are completely unreasonable in view of the task demands. Unreasonable solutions also appear on questions for which there is some evidence that the child understands the procedure. In other instances, such children fail to generate a reasonable plan of action when the requirements of a particular mechanical arithmetic question are only slightly different from procedures that the child has obviously mastered. This failure to generalize a particular skill so that it can be adapted to a new, slightly different situation is a predominant feature of the general adaptational characteristics of these children.

These aspects of the mechanical arithmetic performance of group A children would appear to be qualitative reflections of (1) their difficulties in visual-spatial-organizational and psychomotor skills and concept-formation and hypothesis-testing abilities and (2) their adequate verbal memory skills, which fail due to shortcomings in their capacity to deploy such skills adaptively because of difficulties in understanding when particular bits of stored information are needed during the course of a calculation procedure. Some of these types of mechanical arithmetic errors can be found in the profiles of other arithmetic-impaired children who exhibit types and degrees of neuropsychological deficiencies that are somewhat different from those of children in group A. However, many of the foregoing characteristics (especially regarding errors that result from deficient judgment and reasoning) distinguish group A children from their (nonmentally retarded) agemates.

Studies 7 and 8

Among our most recent studies are two that have employed almost all of the aforementioned measures in an investigation of groups 1 (R-S-A), 2 (R-S), and 3 (A) learning-disabled children between the ages of 7 and 8 years (Ozols & Rourke, 1988, in press). These yielded results in the case of verbal, auditory-perceptual, and visual-spatial skills and abilities that were quite comparable with those obtained in study 4 with 9- to 14-year-old children (Rourke & Finlayson, 1978). However, as in study 3 (Rourke, Dietrich, & Young, 1973), where 6- to 8-year-old children were assigned to groups on the basis of their patterns of WISC VIQ–PIQ discrepancies, the results were not as clear-cut as were those for the older learning-disabled children of study 5, especially in the areas of motor, psychomotor, and tactile-perceptual skills (Rourke & Strang, 1978). In addition, it was not possible to measure higher-order (formal) reasoning and concept-formation abilities in an adequate fashion in these younger children, who are, in Piaget's terms, still functioning within the stage of concrete operational thought.

Conclusions: Studies 4 through 8

This completes our survey of the levels and configurations of neuropsychological abilities and deficits exhibited by subtypes of learning-disabled children classified on the basis of their patterns of academic performance in reading, spelling, and arithmetic. (For a summary of validation studies of these subtype comparisons from other laboratories, the interested reader is referred to Fletcher, 1985.) On the basis of the results of this program of research, the following general and specific conclusions appear warranted.

General

1. There would appear to be reliable (internally valid) subtypes of learning-disabled children that can be designated on the basis of patterns of academic achievement.

2. These subtypes can be differentiated on neuropsychological variables not employed in the initial classification; that is, the subtypes have external validity.

3. There are some similarities and differences between older (i.e., 9- to 14-year-old) and younger (i.e., 7- to 8-year-old) learning-disabled children so classified. That is, there would appear to be significant developmental dimensions to the manifestations of these subtypes of learning disabilities.

4. There are qualitatively distinct "paths" to equivalent levels of impaired performance in mechanical arithmetic. This distinctness would appear to be a function of the patterns of neuropsychological abilities and deficits exhibited by children who manifest these "academic" subtypes of learning disabilities.

5. Vastly different forms of intervention would appear necessary for some of these subtypes of learning-disabled youngsters.

Specific Comparisons of Group R-S and Group A

As mentioned earlier, group 1 (R-S-A) is probably composed of several different subtypes of learning-disabled children (Petrauskas & Rourke, 1979). It is also the case that the principal neuropsychological comparisons of immediate interest in connection with the NLD syndrome are those between group R-S and group A. Based upon the foregoing analyses, there are several specific conclusions that apply to these two groups. (In the following, "older" refers to 9- to 14-year-old children, "younger" to 7- and 8-year-old children.)

1. Older group R-S children exhibit some (often no more than mild) deficiencies in the more rote aspects of psycholinguistic skills, such as the recall of information and word definitions; older group A children exhibit average to superior skills in these areas.

2. Older group R-S children exhibit outstanding deficiencies in the more complex semantic-acoustic aspects of psycholinguistic skills, such as sentence memory and auditory analysis of common words. Older group A children exhibit less than normal performance in these areas, but their levels of performance are superior to those of group R-S agemates. Older group A children tend to perform least well on those tests of semantic-acoustic processing that place an emphasis upon the processing of novel, complex, and/or meaningful material.

3. Older group R-S children exhibit normal levels of performance on visual-spatial-organizational, psychomotor, and tactile-perceptual

tasks; older group A children have outstanding difficulties on such tasks. The deficiencies exhibited by older group A children on tactile-perceptual and psychomotor tasks are in evidence bilaterally; when there is evidence of lateralized impairment on such tasks for the group A child, it is almost always a relative deficiency in performance on the left side of the body. In general, the more novel the visual-spatial, psychomotor, and tactile-perceptual task, the more impairment, relative to age-based norms, is evident in the older group A child's performance.

4. Older group R-S children perform normally on nonverbal problem-solving tasks. They have no difficulty in benefiting from experience with such tasks. They are particularly adept at utilizing nonverbal informational feedback in order to modify their performance to meet the demands of such tasks. Older group A children exhibit profound problems on nonverbal problem-solving tasks. They give little or no evidence of benefiting from informational feedback and continued experience with such tasks, even when the information provided would be expected to be well within their reach, based upon their rote verbal learning capacity (e.g., Verbal IQ).

5. Younger group R-S and group A children exhibit inter- and intragroup patterns of relative abilities and deficits on automatic (rote) verbal, semantic-acoustic, and visual-spatial-organizational tasks that are similar to those exhibited by older children in these two groups. The exception is that the more rote aspects of verbal skills tend to be more deficient relative to age-based norms in younger than in older group R-S children.

6. Differentiations in terms of psychomotor and tactile-perceptual skills and abilities are far less marked in younger than in older children of these two groups.

7. Although there is some evidence to suggest that younger group A children have more difficulty in adapting to novel problem-solving situations than do their group R-S counterparts, the precise measurement of such suspected difficulties has yet to be completed.

Note on Research Methodology. These conclusions and generalizations should be sufficient to make the desired point, namely, that learning-disabled children chosen solely *on the basis of specific variations in patterns of academic performance (with adequate controls for age, Full Scale IQ, and other important attributes) can be shown to exhibit very different patterns of neuropsychological abilities and deficits. In this connection, it should be noted that both of the subtypes under considera-*

tion exhibited deficient mechanical arithmetic performance. Thus, members of each of these groups could have been included in the "learning-disabled" sample of a contrasting-groups type of study that was designed to compare "arithmetic-disabled" and "normal" children. It should be clear, from the preceding conclusions and generalizations, that such an "arithmetic-disabled" group could be made up of at least two very distinct arithmetic-disabled subtypes. It is also the case that (1) these subtypes of children share virtually nothing in common, from a neuropsychological standpoint, (2) their similarly deficient levels of performance in mechanical arithmetic reflect these quite different "etiologies," and (3) their needs for academic habilitation/rehabilitation with respect to mechanical arithmetic differ markedly from one another. See Rourke and Strang (1983), Strang and Rourke (1985a, 1985b), and subsequent chapters of this book for a discussion of these issues.

Although not evident in the results of the studies reviewed to this point, it appears to be the case that the adaptive implications of the relative abilities and deficits of older group R-S and group A children extend well beyond the confines of the academic setting. For example, group R-S children tend to fare far better in social situations than do group A children. More precise delineations of these extra-academic learning considerations are presented later in this book.

STATISTICAL DERIVATION AND PHONETIC ACCURACY OF MISSPELLINGS

We turn now to a consideration of two other classes of learning-disabilities investigations that have been carried out in our laboratory, parallel to those just discussed. These studies have some relevance for the NLD model, which is the principal focus of inquiry of this work. They are reviewed only briefly because, although important, they are not entirely pivotal to the understanding of this model.

Statistically Derived Subtypes

The studies reviewed to this point would certainly suggest that disabled learners do not constitute a homogeneous group. Two studies conducted in our laboratory that dealt specifically with disabled readers and "across-the-board" learning-disabled youngsters (Fisk & Rourke, 1979; Petrauskas & Rourke, 1979) would serve to bolster this contention. The results of these investigations are important with respect to the NLD model in that they suggest that it is possible to isolate functions of a linguistic nature, and that these isolatable functions appear to be related to different subtypes of disabled reading. The results of these studies are also relevant to the larger issues concerning the definition of learning disabilities and investigative strategies for research in the neuropsychology of learning disabilities, which are discussed in Chapter 8.

The Petrauskas and Rourke (1979) study involved the classification of disabled readers between the ages of 7.0 and 8.9 years by means of the technique of Q factor analysis. Three reliable subtypes of retarded readers were found at this age level, and a fourth subtype was delineated that was composed primarily of normal readers. It was also found that the three subtypes of retarded readers that were isolated were rather similar to subtypes of disabled readers that had been suggested in the clinical literature (Mattis, French, & Rapin, 1975).

In a cross-sectional investigation of 9- to 14-year-old learning-disabled children who exhibited scores below the 30th centile on the Reading, Spelling, and Arithmetic subtests of the WRAT (Fisk & Rourke, 1979), we were particularly interested in whether any identified subtypes would persist over time. From the total sample of subjects, three subsamples that were based on 2-year age intervals were composed, and each age-based sample was equated for WISC Full Scale IQ.

Each age-based sample was subjected to a separate Q factor analysis; this yielded a classification of 80% of the learning-disabled children at the three age levels. The most interesting aspect of this study was that two of these subtypes were found at all three age levels, and a third was in evidence at the two older age levels. The correlations *among* the subtypes that were replicated across age levels were, by definition, very high (in the 80s and 90s), as were the visual configurations for each of their sets of scores on the 21 variables employed in the study. Of particular interest was the fact that the correlations *between* the three subtypes that were replicated across either two or three of the age levels were nonsignificant. This would certainly suggest that these replicated subtypes of disabled readers are quite independent of one another, and that they represent very stable configurations of neuropsychological abilities and deficits that tend to persist across the age span from 9 to 14 years.

The stability of these subtypes is of particular interest with respect to the NLD model, since one of its principal foundations involves stability and change within a particular subtype of learning-disabled person throughout the course of development. In this connection, a recent study by Morris, Blashfield, and Satz (1986) is an excellent illustration of change and stability in subtypes of disabled readers studied within the context of a longitudinal design.

Phonetic Accuracy of Misspellings

In a series of studies (Sweeney & Rourke, 1978, 1985; Rourke & Russell, 1989; Russell & Rourke, 1989; Russell, Rourke, & Knights, 1989), we have examined the neuropsychological significance of levels of phonetic accuracy of misspellings among disabled spellers and readers. These studies were prompted by the oft-noted observation of the pattern of language recovery in adults following significant craniocerebral trauma and other types of neurological disease. Specifically, we were impressed by the observation that the persistence of phonetically inaccurate misspellings, during late periods of recovery from the aphasia that resulted from the neurological disease in question, is associated with long-term linguistic disability.

In order to carry out these studies, we developed a method for scoring, on a syllable-by-syllable basis, the level of phonetic accuracy of misspellings (Sweeney & Rourke, 1978). Two sets of studies (Sweeney & Rourke, 1978, 1985) employed disabled spellers who were equated for level of spelling but who differed markedly in the levels of phonetic accuracy of their misspellings. These subtypes of learning-disabled children were dubbed, as might be expected, "phonetically accurate" and "phonetically inaccurate" disabled spellers. Two other studies in this series (Rourke & Russell, 1989; Russell & Rourke, 1989; Russell et al., 1989) took a somewhat different tack: They involved considerations of normal and disabled spellers and readers where phonetic accuracy of misspellings was treated as a continuous variable. The results of these studies led to the following conclusions:

1. There are reliable subtypes of disabled learners that can be differentiated in terms of level of phonetic accuracy of misspellings.
2. There are significant developmental dimensions in the manifestations of subtypes of children identified on this basis.
3. Children classified as "phonetically accurate" and "phonetically inaccurate" disabled spellers would appear to require quite differ-

ent modes of intervention in order to enhance their progress in the academic milieu.

4. Level of phonetic accuracy of misspellings is a powerful predictor of (a) neuropsychological status (concurrent validity) on variables outside of the realm of psycholinguistic functioning and (b) future levels of academic skill development (predictive validity).

These findings are important for the development of an understanding of the NLD syndrome. As pointed out in the brief description of the model presented in Chapter 1, children who exhibit NLD develop considerable expertise in producing phonetically accurate reproductions of words delivered by oral dictation. Indeed, their level of accuracy is much greater than that exhibited by "normal" spellers. This "hyperphonetic" accuracy is an especially relevant dimension to appreciate in such children, because it reflects a more general proclivity for an overdependence upon auditory—as opposed to visual or tactile—stimuli in their perceptual repertoires.

Having discussed the evidence for the existence of learning disability subtypes, we turn in the next chapter to a consideration of studies dealing with the socioemotional and adaptive dimensions of learning disabilities in children. These factors are believed to be intimately related to considerations of subtypes as discussed in this chapter, an assumption that is integral to the NLD syndrome and model presented in Chapters 5 and 6.

CHAPTER THREE

Socioemotional Disturbances of Learning-Disabled Children

This chapter is designed to evaluate support for one minor and two major hypotheses regarding the relationships between socioemotional disturbance and learning disabilities in children and adolescents (see Table 3.1). Some evidence regarding these relationships in adults is also presented. Although the principal focus in this chapter is on those studies conducted in our laboratory that served to feed into the development of the NLD syndrome, it is necessary to carry out a brief review of some other research in this area in order to provide the mise-en-scène for the discussion of these interrelated investigations.

The role of socioemotional disturbance in the etiology and consequences of childhood learning disabilities has been studied extensively over the past quarter of a century. In order to focus our inquiry in this area, I thought it advisable to frame it in terms of the principal questions that this examination is designed to answer. It should come as no surprise that these questions are those that are particularly germane to the formulation and explication of the NLD syndrome and model. The questions of interest are as follows:

- Do learning-disabled children suffer from mild to severe forms of socioemotional disturbance more often than do other children?
- Is there a particular pattern of emotional disturbance or social incompetence displayed by learning-disabled children?
- Are there distinct types of socioemotional disturbance exhibited by learning-disabled children?
- If so, are these more frequent in such children than in their normally achieving peers?
- Is there any particular pattern of central processing abilities and deficits that leads both to a particular configuration of academic achievement in word recognition, spelling, and arithmetic and to a particular form of socioemotional disturbance?

TABLE 3.1. Three Hypotheses Addressing the Relationships between
Socioemotional Disturbance and Learning Disabilities

Hypothesis 1: Socioemotional disturbance causes learning disabilities.

Hypothesis 2: Learning disabilities cause socioemotional disturbance and deficiencies in
social competence.

Hypothesis 3: Specific patterns of central processing abilities and deficits cause specific
manifestations (subtypes) of learning disabilities and specific forms of socioemotional
disturbance and deficiencies in social competence.

- Are there other patterns of central processing abilities and deficits
  that lead to particular configurations of academic achievement but
  not to predictable patterns of socioemotional disturbance?
- Is there evidence to suggest that learning-disabled youngsters, as a
  group, tend to become more prone to socioemotional disturbance
  with advancing years?
- Is there any particular subtype of learning-disabled child that is
  prone to worsening of the manifestations of psychopathology with
  advancing years?

*Note on Format. In the following, as in Chapter 2, those investigations
carried out in our laboratory are numbered (study 1, 2, 3, etc.), in order
to distinguish them from the flow of the review in which they are
embedded. These numbers do not refer to the same studies so numbered
in Chapter 2, however.*

HYPOTHESIS 1

Before dealing with the two major hypotheses that are the focus of
concern in this chapter, another widely held position should be raised
and dealt with, specifically, the notion that socioemotional disturbance
causes learning disabilities. In this view, learning problems that children
face in school and elsewhere are thought to constitute one reflection of
systematic disturbances in socioemotional functioning (e.g., unresolved
psychic conflicts). The evidence for this assertion arises from a variety of
sources, mostly "clinical" in nature.

For example, it has been observed by many whose professional work
brings them into contact with youngsters who are experiencing problems

in academic learning that a significant proportion, if not most, of these children suffer from one or more difficulties of a socioemotional sort. These include personality conflicts with their teachers that render learning in the classroom difficult, if not impossible; strain associated with difficulties in meeting the perceived demands (often exaggerated) of their parents and teachers; extreme psychic conflicts that render them almost incapable of benefiting from ordinary scholastic instruction; and motivation for academic success that is "inappropriate" and social expectancies that are at variance with those of the school (Rourke, Bakker, Fisk, & Strang, 1983; Rourke, Fisk, & Strang, 1986). These examples illustrate that social conflict between teacher and student should be kept to a minimum if academic learning is to proceed apace; that unrealistic ego ideals can, and usually do, have a profound negative impact on performance; that significant intrapsychic conflicts, no matter how generated and maintained, can impact significantly on academic performance; and that the school is largely a middle-class institution that requires at least the temporary adoption of its standards (in North America, largely those of the Protestant Ethic) for success in its programs.

These few examples should serve to illustrate the enormous number of complex sets of interactions that can serve to limit significantly the academic progress of untold numbers of students. In all of these instances, the socioemotional "problem" antedates the difficulty in academic learning; this is so even in the case of teacher–student conflict. Furthermore, it is assumed by most observers that, were the socioemotional problems to be resolved, satisfactory academic performance would ensue. Thus, solving the student–teacher personality conflicts, bringing ego ideals more closely in tune with reality, rectifying the intrapsychic conflict, and leading the student to adopt a motivational posture and social-expectancy set that are more in line with those of the school would be expected to lead eventually to satisfactory academic progress.

This having been said, it is also necessary to point out that these matters really have to do with an etiology for academic and other learning difficulties that is usually excluded under the widely accepted definition of learning disability. In the traditional view, persons are designated learning disabled if their significant problems in learning are *not* a result of primary emotional disturbance (or mental retardation, primary sensory handicap, inadequate instruction, inappropriate motivation, or cultural/linguistic deprivation). Thus, although interesting in and of themselves, and of obvious importance for the total understanding and treatment of children's problems in learning, these factors are not usually considered within the context of socioemotional correlates of this particular definition of learning *disability*.

The remainder of this chapter is devoted to a consideration of studies that ostensibly have employed such exclusionary definitions of learning disabilities. As is pointed out in subsequent chapters of this work, however, the particular constraints vis-à-vis mental retardation, frank brain damage, and other factors such as socioemotional disturbance that have been placed upon considerations germane to the neuropsychological investigation of learning disabilities are, in my view, of limited current relevance.

HYPOTHESIS 2

The second hypothesis is the first of major interest within the present context and is one that, as in the aforementioned view, proposes a causal link between learning difficulties and socioemotional disturbance (Rourke & Fisk, 1981). The differences in this instance are that (1) learning disability, as commonly defined (Rourke, 1975), is the focus of interest; and (2) the causal relationship is reversed; that is, it is proposed that learning disabilities lead to emotional disturbance. This proposition has a very compelling, tacit appeal for most clinicians; it concretizes a view that is widely held and has become almost a cornerstone of clinical lore in this area.

The reasons for the *prima facie* appeal of this view are numerous. For example, it appears to make good clinical sense to maintain that a learning-disabled youngster who persists in having learning problems throughout the elementary school year will be the butt of criticism and negative evaluations by parents, teachers, and agemates; that these criticisms will serve to render the learning-disabled child more anxious and less self-assured in learning situations; that a vicious circle will develop which increasingly hampers academic success and encourages progressively more debilitating degrees of anxiety (i.e., learning failure → increased anxiety → feelings of inferiority → learning failure, and so on); and that this sort of undesirable situation is virtually inevitable and would be expected to increase in severity as the child fails to make advances in academic learning. It would be instructive to examine some of the research that has been viewed as support for this position.

Emotional Disturbance

Review and Critique of the Literature

This research has focused on the emotional, social, and behavioral functioning of learning-disabled children, particularly with respect to their interpersonal environments. For example, investigators have examined characteristics of learning-disabled children's parents (Goldman & Barclay, 1974; Grunebaum, Hurwitz, Prentice, & Sperry, 1962; Wetter, 1972) and the communication patterns within these families (Campbell, 1972; Miller & Westman, 1964; Peck & Stackhouse, 1973). Also, the manner in which learning-disabled children have been perceived by their parents (e.g., Seigler & Gynther, 1960; Stag, 1972), by teachers (e.g., Bryan & McGrady, 1972; McCarthy & Paraskevopoulos, 1969), by peers (e.g., Bryan, 1974b, 1976; Sipperstein, Bopp, & Bak, 1978), and by independent observers (e.g., Bryan, 1974a; Richey & McKinney, 1978) has been examined.

This literature would appear to suggest that learning-disabled children must deal with interpersonal environments that differ markedly from those that confront their normally achieving peers. In contrast to normal achievers, learning-disabled children are (1) perceived as less pleasant and desirable by parents, teachers, and peers; (2) the recipients of more negative communications from their parents, teachers, and peers; (3) ignored and rejected more often by their teachers; (4) treated in a notably more punitive and derogatory manner by their parents; and (5) likely to live in families that resemble in important ways those of emotionally disturbed children. Indeed, it is widely held that learning-disabled children are particularly prone to socioemotional difficulties (Connolly, 1971; Natchez, 1968). Some investigators have even suggested that a particular pattern of socioemotional problems is generally descriptive of the learning-disabled child (e.g., Black, 1974; Halechko, 1977; Zimmerman & Allebrand, 1965).

This hypothesized relationship between learning disabilities and socioemotional disturbance has been assessed directly in a few reasonably controlled studies, which have contrasted groups of learning-disabled children with groups of normally achieving peers. For example, McNutt (1978) found learning-disabled adolescents to be more poorly adjusted both emotionally and socially than their normally achieved agemates; Zimmerman and Allebrand (1965) found more emotional maladjustment among learning-disabled children, but rough comparability of the two groups on almost every measure of social adjustment; and Connolly (1969) found no between-group differences regarding either personality organization or degree of emotional disturbance. A similar degree of inconsistency of results is evident in studies of self-esteem in learning-disabled youngsters: Halechko (1977) and Black (1974) found lower self-esteem among learning-disabled children, whereas Silverman (1978), using the same instrument as did Black, found no between-group differences. Ribner (1978) found that normal achievers demonstrated greater self-esteem than as-yet-undiagnosed learning-disabled children in regular classrooms, but that identified learning-disabled children in segregated classes could not be distinguished from normal achievers on the basis of self-esteem.

Problems similar to those noted in connection with the comparative-populations or contrasting-groups methodologies in the field of learning disabilities more generally (see Chapter 1) are relevant here. On the whole, this research relating to the presumed psychopathological correlates of learning disabilities in children has not been terribly contributory. For example, the results of many studies are trivial, contradictory to one another, and not supported in replication attempts; there is little to suggest that the emotional factors identified as characteristic of learning-disabled children in these studies are related to one another in any meaningful fashion. In sum, the evidence regarding socioemotional functioning that emerges from the research is, at best, equivocal. A coherent and meaningful pattern of personality characteristics of children with learning disabilities does not emerge, which may very well be the case because, as already proposed, the assumption of a univocal pattern does not obtain. (More will be said on this point later.)

More basic problems with such research are as follows:

1. *Definition of Learning Disabilities.* There is no consistent formulation of the criteria for learning disabilities in these studies.

2. *Measurement of Maladjustment.* The concepts of "emotional disturbance," "socioemotional adjustment," "personality characteristics," and "disturbed pattern of family functioning" have been operationalized as inadequately (or perhaps more so) than has "learning disability" in many of these studies. It is clear that the use of reliable and valid psychometric instruments would be preferable to the largely subjective nature of the judgments made about these crucial dependent variables.

3. *Developmental Considerations.* Several studies offer support for the notion that the nature of the skill and ability deficits of some subtypes

of learning-disabled children varies with age (e.g., McKinney et al., 1985; Morris et al., 1986; Ozols & Rourke, 1988; Rourke, Dietrich, & Young, 1973). Since it would seem reasonable to infer that the socioemotional functioning of (some subtypes of) learning-disabled children would also vary as a function of age (considered as one index of developmental change), the inconsistencies in research results could reflect differences in the ages of the subjects employed. To investigate this possibility, cross-sectional or longitudinal studies, such as that carried out by Peter and Spreen (1979), are necessary. (See below for other examples of such an approach in this area of investigation.)

4. *Heterogeneity*. Virtually all of the studies mentioned have employed a research design that involves comparisons of undifferentiated groups of learning-disabled children to equally undifferentiated groups of normal achievers. This approach, which aims to identify *the particular pattern* of socioemotional disturbance of learning-disabled children tends to obscure within-group differences. As Applebee (1971) has pointed out, employment of this comparative-populations approach can only be justified if one can safely assume that learning-disabled children are homogeneous in terms of their abilities and deficits. As I have contended in earlier chapters, recent neuropsychological research has suggested strongly that these children constitute a heterogeneous population in terms of their skills and abilities and that meaningful subtypes of learning-disabled children can be identified in a reliable fashion (e.g., Fletcher, 1985; Morris et al., 1981; Rourke & Adams, 1984; Rourke & Finlayson, 1978; Rourke & Strang, 1978; Strang & Rourke, 1983). It is also the case that this heterogeneity is evident in the socioemotional functioning of these children, as demonstrated in the results of the following studies.

Studies 1, 2, and 3

In an attempt to examine the heterogeneity hypothesis, we selected 100 learning-disabled children between the ages of 5 and 15 for study 1 (Porter & Rourke, 1985). These subjects met the usual exclusionary criteria that have been utilized in the vast majority of our previous investigations (Rourke, 1975, 1978b). In this study, the Q factor analysis algorithm was employed to analyze the clinical scales of the Personality Inventory for Children (PIC), a measure that has been subjected to fairly extensive reliability and validity studies with good to excellent results (Wirt, Lachar, Klinedinst, & Seat, 1977).

As a first step in the analysis of these data, the mean PIC profile for the total sample of 100 subjects was generated. It revealed that the Intellectual Screening scale was significantly elevated (T score > 70) and that only the Achievement scale approached this level. These scale elevations, which revealed deviations in the direction of increased parental concern about or perception of school achievement or cognitive difficulties, would be expected in any sample of learning-disabled children. The clinical scales specifically designed to evaluate socioemotional functioning were within normal limits. At this point in the data analysis of this study, the results would suggest that learning-disabled children are not particularly prone to socioemotional difficulties; however, the results of the subsequent Q factor analysis of the PIC data suggested a very different interpretation. It revealed that 77 of the 100 subjects could be classified into four socioemotional subtypes; multivariate analyses of variance revealed significant differences across the four subtypes overall as well as on 28 of the 33 individual PIC scales. The following analysis of the results of this subtype analysis is germane to the issues raised in this section.

The largest subtype identified (made up of approximately 50% of the classified subjects) showed no indications of any elevations on the scales reflecting socioemotional disturbance; that is, the children were rated as well adjusted in terms of their socioemotional functioning. A second subtype (approximately 25% of those classified) exhibited a PIC profile suggestive of seriously disturbed socioemotional functioning of the internalized variety, marked by such dimensions as depression, withdrawal, and anxiety. The third subtype (approximately 15% of those classified) was characterized by scale elevations typically seen in children diagnosed as "hyperkinetic," a disorder usually manifest in externalized dimensions such as aggressiveness. This particular profile was virtually identical to that reported by Breen and Barkley (1984) in their investigation of the PIC profiles of "hyperactive" children. A fourth subtype (approximately 10% of the classified subjects) exhibited roughly normal socioemotional functioning accompanied by a variety of somatic complaints; that is, their only significantly elevated clinical scale was Somatic Concern.

A subsequent analysis (study 2) of these four subtypes using PIC factor scales instead of individual T scores revealed that the first ("normal") and fourth ("somatic concern") subtypes could not be differentiated on the basis of stepwise discriminant function analysis (Rourke, Pohlman, Fuerst, Porter, & Fisk, 1985). Hence, it would appear that there are *three* replicable socioemotional subtypes of learning-disabled youngsters in this data base.

A recent third study (Fuerst, Fisk, & Rourke, 1989a) carried out in our laboratory confirms and expands this three-subtype finding; that is, there would appear to be three socioemotional subtypes of learning-disabled children, classified as "normal," "emotionally disturbed," and "hyperactive."

There were no significant age differences between the PIC-generated subtypes in the Porter and Rourke (1985) and Rourke, Pohlman, et al. (1985) studies. Strang (1981) also found no indication of any increased incidence of psychopathology (as measured with the PIC) over cross-sectional comparisons of undifferentiated groups of learning-disabled children between the ages of 8 and 12 years. These results contrast sharply with suggestions of increased incidence of psychopathology in learning-disabled children over this age span (Lorin, Cowen, & Caldwell, 1974; Routh & Mesibov, 1980).

Studies by McKinney and Colleagues

An interesting series of studies by McKinney and his colleagues is also of considerable interest within this context. Speece, McKinney, and Appelbaum (1985) were able to classify 63 school-identified learning-disabled children (average age approximately 7 years) into seven "behavioral" subtypes by means of one type of cluster analysis. The Classroom Behavior Inventory (CBI; Schaefer, Edgerton, & Aronson, 1977), a rating instrument completed by classroom teachers, was the measure used for clustering. These investigators went to some lengths to examine the internal validity (reliability) and external validity of the subtypes generated. In addition to demonstrating that these behavioral learning-disabled subtypes were different from one another, they showed that the profile patterns generated were quite different from those evident among normally achieving controls. Yet it was also the case that approximately one-third of the learning-disabled children who were classified exhibited profiles on the CBI that were completely normal. Some of the other subtypes generated also exhibited profiles that were, at most, within the borderline or very mildly impaired range. It was also the case that subtypes characterized by conduct disorder, withdrawn behavior, and fairly serious, global behavior problems were isolated. These normal and deviant behavioral subtypes bear a strong resemblance to those isolated by Porter and Rourke (1985) and Rourke et al. (1985). A 3-year longitudinal follow-up of 47 of these youngsters (McKinney & Speece, 1986) yielded evidence of some stability of the subtypes and some change in subtype membership over time. Of interest was the finding that the subtype membership change for the learning-disabled children was very clearly from one "pathological" group to another, rather than to the normal subtype patterns.

Except for the use of a criterion for the determination of learning disability that is difficult to verify or replicate, and some questionable re-groupings of the behavioral subtypes in the longitudinal phases, these studies are marked by a degree of care and precision that contitutes an important contribution to the testing of the hypothesis under consideration.

Conclusions

The results of these studies of emotional disturbance constitute a formidable challenge to the view that learning-disabled children are relatively uniform in terms of their socioemotional functioning. Furthermore, they cast doubt on the notion that learning disability, broadly considered, constitutes a sufficient condition for the production of emotional disturbance. Put simply, the results of these studies suggest strongly that some children who meet commonly accepted (i.e., traditional or exclusionary) criteria for learning disability show signs of significant socioemotional disturbance, whereas others do not; on balance, it appears that most do not. The important question at this juncture becomes one of determining whether there is a set of characteristics that differentiates learning-disabled youngsters who develop adaptive socioemotional coping patterns from those who develop internalized or externalized forms of socioemotional disturbance. This issue is taken up in the discussion of hypothesis 3, in the context of an explanation of the relationship between neuropsychological skill/ability patterns and socioemotional disturbance.

Social Competence

Review and Critique of the Literature

With the context of the consideration of hypothesis 2, we turn to a review of some research dealing with the social competence of learning-disabled youngsters. This area of investigation dovetails rather well with the series of studies on socioemotional functioning just outlined and with those that are considered in conjunction with hypothesis 3. Dimensions of social competence are also crucial considerations in the NLD syndrome.

As was seen to be the case with the investigations of socioemotional disturbance, the experimental hypothesis most often tested in this area is that of a causal link between learning disabilities and social competence, specifically, that learning disabilities lead to deficiencies in social competence.

Social competence may be conceptualized as a child's ability to satisfy interpersonal needs in ways that are both effective and acceptable to society. The importance of the study of this dimension in learning-disabled children is highlighted by evidence that adult mental health is correlated with childhood social competence (Cowen, Pederson, Babigian, Izzo, & Trost, 1973). Social competence is difficult to define in operational terms, and researchers interested in determining characteristics of socially competent children (e.g., Nakamura & Finck, 1980) acknowledge the variability of effective social behavior and recognize the importance of situational determinants of such behavior. Nevertheless, the component analysis of effective social functioning (e.g., Anderson & Messick, 1974) appears to have considerable heuristic value. For example, the large number of skills and abilities identified by a component analysis of social competence can be classified into three groups: (1) perceptual skills, such as those needed for the perception of facial expressions; (2) cognitive abilities, such as those required to discern cause-and-effect relationships in social events; and (3) motor and language skills, by which children manifest their social behavior. Competent social behavior can be seen as a result of a complex interaction and coordination of these and related variables. It is also widely held that attitudinal characteristics (e.g., differentiated self-concept and consolidation of identity, a concept of oneself as an initiating and controlling agent, and a realistic appraisal of oneself, accompanied by feelings of personal worth) are crucial factors in the development of social competence.

Literature in this area reveals frequent claims that learning-disabled children experience problems in their social relationships, and that their socioemotional difficulties persist into adolescence and adulthood (Bryan, Donohue, & Pearl, 1981; Kronick, 1980; Siegel, 1974). Variables that have been utilized to investigate the validity of such claims include parent observations (Owen, Adams, Forrest, Stolz, & Fisher, 1971), teacher ratings (Bryan & McGrady, 1972; Keogh, Tchir, & Windeguth-Behn, 1974), peer ratings (Bryan, 1974b), classroom observations of the interactions of learning-disabled students (Bryan, 1974a; Bryan & Wheeler, 1972), and behavior checklists (McConaughty & Ritter, 1986).

The results of these studies have demonstrated consistently that, in comparison to their normally achieving peers, learning-disabled young-sters tend to be judged in more negative and rejecting terms by parents, teachers, and classmates, and/or that they are perceived as much less competent in social adaptation. Such comparisons have also shown that some learning-disabled children are relatively deficient in perceiving their own social status (Bruininks, 1978).

Explanations for these deficiencies have usually focused on a *single* perceptual, cognitive, or behavioral skill that is said to be lacking in learning-disabled children—for example, a schematic judgment deficit, or an inability to realize the organization of an interactional situation (Kronick, 1980); or a linguistic deficit that results in poor interpersonal communication skills and problems in understanding the rules that govern socially appropriate speech (Bryan, 1982).

Some studies have examined the learning-disabled child's ability to perceive and interpret accurately the affective states of others. Deficiencies in labeling emotions expressed through nonverbal means (Wiig & Harris, 1974), selecting appropriate facial expressions for material presented in stories (Bachara, 1976), and describing emotional scenarios from videotaped displays of emotion (Bryan, 1977) have been documented.

Analogous to the problems noted in Chapter 1 with respect to the contrasting-groups methodology, there would appear to be at least two major reasons why the results of these studies of social competence are not very contributory to the testing of hypothesis 2. Elements of each of these are alluded to by La Greca (1981).

1. Lack of a Conceptual Model. There is an obvious absence in these studies of a conceptual model for elucidating the skills involved in social competence, which are presumably deficient in learning-disabled children. (A notable exception to this is the formulation of Wiener, 1980.) For example, at the very minimum, a component analysis of social competence should sensitize the researcher to the possibility that, whereas some subtypes of learning-disabled children may experience social competence problems because they lack certain perceptual, cognitive, or behavioral skills, others may manifest such problems as a more direct result of attitudinal/motivational difficulties. It should also be clear that different patterns of perceptual, cognitive, and behavioral skills and abilities may encourage different types of degrees of socially incompetent behavior.

2. Definitional Problems and Subtypes. Related to the first problem is the use of inconsistent and/or unclear definitions of learning disabilities in these studies, and an almost total lack of sensitivity to the notion that there may be subtypes of learning-disabled children for whom various types of social competence may be more or less difficult to achieve. A notable exception to the latter problem is the work of McConaughty and Ritter (1986).

Study 4

An example of research that has attempted to grapple with some of the difficulties presented by the approaches just reviewed is the investigation by Ozols and Rourke (1985), involving two groups of learning-disabled children. The first was an R-S group (see Chapter 2), whose members exhibited many relatively poor psycholinguistic skills in conjunction with very well-developed abilities in visual-spatial-organizational, tactile-perceptual, psychomotor, and nonverbal problem-solving skills. They also experienced very poor reading and spelling skills and significantly better, though still impaired, mechanical arithmetic competence. The second group was of the group A type (also described in Chapter 2). These children exhibited outstanding problems in visual-spatial-organizational, tactile-perceptual, psychomotor, and nonverbal problem-solving skills, within a context of clear strengths in some psycholinguistic skills such as rote verbal learning, regular phoneme–grapheme matching, amount of verbal output, and verbal classification. Group A children experienced their major academic learning difficulties in mechanical arithmetic, while exhibiting advanced levels of word-recognition and spelling. (As will be seen in Chapters 5 and 6, these children are most similar to those with the NLD syndrome.)

The performance of these two groups of learning-disabled children was compared on four exploratory measures of social judgment and responsiveness. One finding was that children in the R-S group performed more effectively than did those in group A on tasks requiring nonverbal responses; in contrast, tasks requiring verbal responses yielded exactly the opposite results. This suggests that social awareness and responsiveness vary markedly for these two subtypes of learning-disabled children, probably as a result of an interaction between their particular patterns of central processing abilities and deficits and the specific task demands of the four measures employed.

The results of the Ozols and Rourke (1985) investigation should be viewed within the context of a study by Ackerman and Howes (1986). In the latter, it was demonstrated that, although social competence deficits often occur in many learning-disabled children, it is the case that some do not exhibit such deficits and are seen as popular with their peers and active in after-school interests. These findings, taken together, would suggest that a study designed along the lines of the Porter and Rourke (1985) investigation may reveal an analogous set of "social competence" subtypes, falling into both "normal" and "disturbed" categories. The studies by Speece et al. (1985) and McKinney and Speece (1986) contain some data that could be used to address this question directly.

Conclusions

It is clear that, as in the case of the investigation of emotional disturbance in learning-disabled youngsters, the examination of their social competence should eschew the homogeneous, contrasting-groups methodology that has heretofore characterized all but a few studies in the field, in favor of one that does justice to the heterogeneity of subtypes evident in the learning-disabled population. Furthermore, it would appear to be the case that efforts to relate patterns of learning abilities and deficits with components of socoemotional development may generate much more interesting data and conclusions than do approaches that simply search for correlates of learning disabilities (considered as a univocal phenomenon) and either emotional disturbance or problems in social competence. The studies reviewed in connection with the examination of hypothesis 3 constitute another step further along the road away from the latter contrasting-groups and unitary-deficit methodologies.

HYPOTHESIS 3

The other major hypothesis that has been investigated in the area of socioemotional disturbance in learning-disabled children proposes a causal connection between (1) particular patterns of central processing abilities and deficits and (2) particular subtypes of learning disabilities and socioemotional functioning (Rourke & Fisk, 1981). The principal data that would suggest support for this hypothesis are, once again, those that arise from a study of group R-S and group A children.

Study 5

For example, when the average PIC profiles of children chosen to approximate the characteristics of these two subtypes of learning-disabled children were compared (Strang & Rourke, 1985a), it was clear that the profile for group A was similar to that exhibited by the "emotionally disturbed" group in study 1 (Porter & Rourke, 1985), whereas the profile for group R-S children was virtually identical to that exhibited by the "normal" group in that study. Additional examination of three factor scores derived from the PIC revealed that the two groups did not differ significantly on the concern over academic achievement but that they differed sharply on the factors of "personality deviance" and "internalized psychopathology." In both of the latter cases, the group A levels of deviation were significantly higher (i.e., more pathological) than were those for group R-S.

These results, considered within the context of the very different patterns of abilities and deficits exhibited by groups R-S and A (see Chapter 2), offer strong support for hypothesis 3. They show that particular patterns of central processing abilities can eventuate in (1) markedly different subtypes of learning disabilities (groups R-S and A) and (2) markedly different patterns of socioemotional functioning (one characterized by normalcy, the other by an internalized form of psychopathology and personality deviance). Since such group results can be deceiving when applied to the individual case, it should be emphasized that there was very little variance evident in the PIC protocols of the children classified into groups R-S and A in these studies. The interested reader may wish to consult case studies of such youngsters in two recent works (Rourke, Bakker, et al., 1983; Rourke, Fisk, & Strang, 1986) for evidence of such consistent differences in socioemotional manifestations. Additional case studies that exemplify the problems of group A (NLD) children are contained in Chapter 7 of this work.

Study 6

Another investigation in this series is instructive in this context. Since, as has been demonstrated in several previous investigations (see Chapter 2 discussion of Rourke, Young, & Flewelling, 1971), WISC VIQ–PIQ discrepancies can serve as a sensitive index of variations in ability structure among learning-disabled youngsters, it was felt that such an index would also be a reasonably sensitive predictor of socioemotional status for such children. To test this hypothesis, Fuerst, Fisk, and Rourke (1989b) did a cluster analysis of PIC data obtained from 132 learning-disabled children between 6 and 12 years of age. Three groups of subjects (22 girls and 22 boys in each group) were equated in a groupwise fashion for age, at two levels of age categorization (6 to 8 years and 9 to 12 years). The subjects within each age category were selected to comprise three equal-sized WISC VIQ–PIQ groups. Thus, there were six groups in all: two HP–LV groups, whose WISC PIQ exceeded VIQ by at least 10 points; two V=P groups, whose WISC VIQ–PIQ discrepancies were no more than 3 points in either direction; and two HV–LP groups, whose WISC VIQ exceeded PIQ by at least 10 points.

The results of the cluster analysis yielded six interpretable clusters, three of which appeared to be virtually identical to those identified in study 1 (Porter & Rourke, 1985)—namely, normal, emotionally disturbed, and hyperactive—and three of which were minor variations of these three. One of the other three clusters that emerged was characterized by scale elevations consistent with those typically seen in children who are considered to be mildly anxious and/or depressed. A fifth appeared to be mildly hyperactive, and a sixth essentially normal. In the present context, the important features of the results of this study relate to the number of subjects from each of the three WISC groupings that loaded within these four PIC clusters. For example, very few of the HV–LP subjects (i.e., those most similar to group A learning-disabled children) were allocated to the "normal" cluster and to the "mild anxiety/depressive" cluster. The subjects comprising the latter clusters were drawn almost exclusively from the V=P and HP–LV subjects (i.e., those most similar to the group R-S learning-disabled children). The HV–LP (group A) subjects constituted a major portion of the "emotionally disturbed" and the "hyperactive" clusters.

In summary, it would appear that children who exhibit the group A (NLD) profile of neuropsychological abilities and deficits are very likely to be described by parents as emotionally or behaviorally disturbed. In contrast, group R-S children (with outstanding difficulties in many aspects of psycholinguistic functioning) are so described at a much lower frequency. More generally, it would appear that the pattern of abilities and deficits exhibited by group A children approximates a sufficient condition for the development of some sort of socioemotional disturbance, whereas the pattern exhibited by group R-S children does not.

This is not meant to imply that children characterized by the group R-S (language-deficient) pattern will never experience socioemotional disturbance. Indeed, clinical experience (e.g., Rourke, Bakker, et al., 1983; Rourke, Fisk, & Strang, 1986) suggests that many do. Rather, these results suggest that, for the group R-S subtype, something *in addition to* psycholinguistic deficiency is necessary for disturbed socioemotional functioning to occur. Such factors may include some of those mentioned in connection with the emotional-disturbance/learning-problem relationship outlined in the initial section of this chapter, such as teacher–pupil personality conflicts, unrealistic demands by parents and teachers, and inappropriate motivation and social expectancies. Others could be the presence of salient antisocial models, selective reinforcement of nonadaptive and socially inappropriate behaviors, and any number of other factors that have the potential for encouraging problems in the socioemotional functioning of even normally achieving youngsters.

Studies 7 and 8

Finally, two studies that were designed to determine the developmental outcome for group A children are germane to the testing of hypothesis 3. Rourke, Young, Strang, and Russell (1986) compared the performance of group A children with that of a group of clinic-referred adults on a wide variety of neuropsychological variables. The adults presented with Wechsler VIQ–PIQ discrepancies and WRAT patterns that were virtually identical to the patterns in group A children. It was demonstrated that the patterns of age-related performance of the adults and the children on the neuropsychological variables were nearly identical. In addition, the adults were characterized by internalized forms of psychopathology that bore a striking resemblance to those exhibited by group A youngsters. In a related study, Del Dotto, Rourke, McFadden, and Fisk (1987) confirmed the stability of the neuropsychological and personality characteristics of the group A children, adolescents, and adults over time.

It is particularly important to note the propensity of the group A (NLD) children to develop a particular configuration of academic learning skills and deficits and a specific type of severe socioemotional disturbance. In the models and the NLD syndrome to be presented in Chapters 4, 5, and 6, the interactions between (1) children's *deficiencies* in neuropsychological dimensions (such as visual-spatial, tactile-perceptual, psychomotor, and concept-formation skills and abilities) and (2) their *excessive reliance upon* one area of strength (specific aspects of language) are characterized as causal vis-à-vis such outcomes. Thus, this interaction and their difficulties in dealing with novel and otherwise complex situations are thought to lie at the root of both sets of adaptive difficulties (i.e., their particular pattern of academic proficiencies and deficiencies and their penchant for a particular form of socioemotional disturbance).

CONCLUSIONS

The principal conclusions and generalizations that have been arrived at on the basis of this inquiry, as they relate to the principal questions posed at the outset of this chapter are as follows:

1. Some learning-disabled children suffer from mild to severe forms of socioemotional disturbance; most appear to experience no such difficulties.

2. There is no single, unitary pattern of emotional disturbance or social incompetence displayed by learning-disabled children.

3. There are distinct types of socioemotional disturbance and behavioral disorder displayed by learning-disabled children. These different manifestations appear to be more frequent among learning-disabled children than among their normally achieving peers.

4. There is at least one pattern of central processing abilities and deficits (that exhibited by group A) that appears to lead both to a particular configuration of academic achievement (well-developed word-recognition and spelling as compared to significantly poorer mechanical arithmetic) and to a particular form of socioemotional disturbance (internalized psychopathology). Other patterns of central processing abilities and deficits (those marked by outstanding difficulties in psycholinguistic skills such as is the case for group R-S) likewise appear to lead to particular patterns of academic achievement (outstanding problems in reading and spelling and varying levels of performance in mechanical arithmetic), with some correlative effect upon the incidence of psychopathology but no particular effect upon its specific manifestations.

5. There is no conclusive evidence to suggest that learning-disabled youngsters, as a group, tend to become more prone to socioemotional disturbance with advancing years. In fact, there is some evidence to suggest that this is not the case.

6. A notable exception to the preceding conclusion is the worsening of the manifestations of psychopathology and the increasing discrepancies between abilities and deficits that are exhibited by children and adolescents of the group A subtype. This is the case in spite of the fact that their *pattern* of neuropsychological abilities and deficits and their

specific manifestations of psychopathology (except for activity level) remain remarkably stable over time.

7. Efforts to clarify the relationships between learning disabilities and socioemotional disturbance should eschew the contrasting-groups/ unitary-deficit approach, in favor of research efforts that deal adequately with the heterogeneity of the learning-disabled population, with respect both to patterns of abilities and deficits and to distinctive forms and manifestations of psychopathology.

There is one additional conclusion that is not matched by a question at the outset of this chapter. This relates to the development of models that are broad and articulated enough to address the complex interactions that take place between (1) patterns of central processing abilities and deficits and (2) academic learning difficulties and socioemotional disturbances. Our review of the literature to this point would lead to the conclusion that continuing to carry out essentially atheoretical, correlational studies of matched groups of learning-disabled and normally achieving children to address the important theoretical and clinical issues in this area is counterproductive. It is clear that models sufficient to deal with the latter (e.g., Fletcher & Taylor, 1984) must be complex and sophisticated.

It is to our own efforts to develop such models that we turn in the next three chapters.

CHAPTER FOUR

The Rourke Right→Left Model (1982)

The first model that was developed to encompass the results of this research enterprise (Rourke, 1982) was designed to provide a context for the interpretation of the conclusions and generalizations outlined in the previous chapters.[1] It was geared particularly to the specification of the interrelationships between socioemotional and adaptive disturbances and manifestations of academic learning difficulties, based on the results of our research program up to that time. It was also meant to provide a heuristic framework for the investigations that would follow. The focus of this model was on developmental and task-related differences and interactions between right- and left-hemisphere systems, hence the "right→left" designation in the title of this chapter.

A general theoretical position (Goldberg & Costa, 1981) was employed as a framework for this neurodevelopmental model of central processing deficiencies in children. While emphasizing differences between right- and left-hemisphere systems, the Rourke (1982) model was designed to embrace a wide variety of behavioral phenomena that have been observed in normal children and in various subtypes of learning-disabled children. It was also designed to address and incorporate dynamic factors operative within the development of both normal and disabled learning.

NEED FOR COMPREHENSIVE MODEL

A complete, unified developmental neuropsychological model of central processing abilities and deficiencies in children should account for (1) the

[1]In order to enhance the reader's appreciation of the role played by the development of the Rourke (1982) model in our research program, most of what follows in this chapter has been cast in the same or very similar terms to the manner in which the model first appeared some 7 years ago.

entire spectrum of children's perceptual, learning, mnestic, and other cognitive abilities and disabilities and (2) the three principal axes of concern in human brain–behavior relationships, namely, the progression from lower to higher centers, that from posterior regions of the cerebrum to the anterior regions, and the right-hemisphere → left-hemisphere progression.

Thus, with respect to the first consideration, a model that is limited to, say, children's problems in learning to read is, simply, quite short of this mark. It is necessary that a complete, unified model be one that can account for children's learning abilities and disabilities in mechanical arithmetic, spelling, social relations, problem solving, and concept formation—in a word, the major dimensions of children's higher-order learning. (At this point, we will exclude consideration of psychomotor learning and lower-order forms of training.)

With respect to encompassing the three dimensions and progressions in neurodevelopment (i.e., down → up, back → front, right → left) these are, of course, oversimplified when stated in this fashion. For example, it is clear that not all lower centers are developed prior to the time that higher systems emerge and mature; that regions of the posterior cerebral cortex (such as the parieto-temporo-occipital area) exhibit myelination well after some areas of frontal cortex (such as the motor strip) have, for all intents and purposes, ceased this process; and that there are those who have held that the progression of cerebral hemispheric organization proceeds from the left to the right hemisphere rather than the other way round (e.g., Corballis & Morgan, 1978).

The vast dimensions of the tasks as thus outlined have encouraged most investigators in this area to confine their theorizing to rather more circumscribed aspects of this domain. Nevertheless, the nature of the problem is not altered: The task remains one of generating a model that is a total, unified explanation of developmental brain–behavior relationships. At the time of the development of the Rourke Right → Left Model (1982), it was not thought possible to provide a comprehensive theory or model that was sufficient for this task. Nevertheless, it was felt desirable to fashion some sort of coherent theoretical structure that would serve at least to explain previous findings and to guide our future research efforts in this area. It was with this goal in mind that this limited model was offered.

The Rourke Right → Left Model (1982) was particularly geared to determining the interrelationships between the development of the brain and the development of the individual's approach to material to be learned. This set of interrelationships constituted the grist for my theoretical mill and was in part based on the assumption that these two "branches" of the brain–behavior relationship, if each were to be better understood, must be investigated within the context of the dynamic interplay of these two types of brain–behavior change. From a statistical standpoint, as well as from a purely notional one, this task implies the necessity for the adoption of multidimensional, multivariate systems of brain–behavior analysis. It will become apparent that such was, indeed is, the case.

While only differences within and between right and left cerebral hemisphere systems and functions were considered, at the same time, it was felt that a fairly broad spectrum of the cognitive dimensions and imperatives could be addressed. Within the context of this constraint on neurodevelopmental dimensions and an attempt to apply this limited perspective to a broad range of higher-order abilities, the model was an attempt to demonstrate that the following principles fit well with much that had been learned to that point from the neuropsychological investigation of central processing abilities—and especially deficiencies—in children:

1. There is an ontogenetic progression from the salience of right-hemisphere functions to that of left-hemisphere functions.
2. The evident change in children's conceptualizations from global to specific is a reflection of this right- to left-hemisphere ontogenetic development.
3. The development of right-hemisphere systems is a prerequisite for the adequate development of left-hemisphere systems.
4. In the normal course of affairs in the formation of constructs and concepts, left-hemisphere systems are particularly geared to their articulation, elaboration, and stereotypic application.
5. Diminished access to or disordered functioning of right-hemisphere systems is especially debilitating with respect to the development of adaptive abilities.

For the most part, these principles and much of this model were drawn from a theoretical position developed by Goldberg and Costa (1981). They propose that the left cerebral hemisphere is more capable of unimodal processing, motor processing, and the storage of compact codes, whereas the right cerebral hemisphere is better suited for intermodal integration, processing of novel stimuli, and dealing with informational complexity. In this conceptualization, the left cerebral hemisphere is viewed as superior in tasks that require fixation on a single mode of representation or execution, and the right cerebral hemisphere is thought to be superior in processing many modes of representation within a single cognitive task.

Since these and related dimensions of the Goldberg and Costa theory of hemispheric differences in the acquisition and use of descriptive systems were crucial for the formulation of this model, a review of selected aspects of this theory is necessary at this juncture.

SELECTED ASPECTS OF THE GOLDBERG AND COSTA MODEL

Goldberg and Costa (1981) point out that there are some significant differences in the cytoarchitecture of the left and right cerebral hemispheres, not the least of which are the opercula (i.e., clumps of grey matter) that are very evident in the temporal, parietal, and posterior frontal regions of the left cerebral hemisphere, and which are not as prominent in the right cerebral hemisphere. Citing cytoarchitectural, neuropsychological, and neurobehavioral evidence from a variety of sources (including Galaburda, LeMay, Kemper, & Geschwind, 1978; Gur et al., 1980; Heilman & Van Den Abell, 1979, 1980; LeMay, 1976; LeMay & Culebras, 1972; Luria, 1966; Wada, Clarke, & Hamm, 1975) that address this and other aspects of differences in left and right hemispheric functioning, Goldberg and Costa (1981) arrived at the following conclusions:

1. For all three main sensory modalities, distinct modality-specific neuronal representations are more prominent in the left hemisphere.
2. Cortical areas of intermodal associative zones are larger in the right hemisphere than in the left hemisphere.
3. The areas of sensory- and motor-specific representations are greater in the left hemisphere, while the right hemisphere is characterized by greater areas of associative cortex.
4. The ratio of grey matter (neuronal mass and short nonmyelinated fibers) to white matter (long myelinated fibers) is higher in the left hemisphere than in the right hemisphere; that is, there is relatively more white matter than grey matter in the right hemisphere than in the left hemisphere.

5. The grey-to-white ratio can be used as a marker of the prevailing organizational feature of a structure in reference to intra- as opposed to interregional integration.
6. There is relatively greater emphasis on interregional integration inherent in the neuronal organization of the right hemisphere, and on intraregional integration in the left hemisphere.
7. The predominantly intraregional pattern of connectivity that characterizes the left hemisphere implies an advantage of the left hemisphere in the processing of simple, unimodal stimuli and in the execution of discrete motor acts.
8. The right hemisphere displays a predominantly interregional pattern of connections. The greater interregional connectivity in the right hemisphere constitutes a greater neuronal capacity to deal with informational complexity.
9. The right hemisphere has a greater ability to process many modes of representation within a single cognitive task, while the left hemisphere is superior in tasks that require fixation upon a single mode of representation or execution.

This model was based primarily upon data gathered and speculations derived from investigations of human adults. Its principal developmental dimension is its emphasis upon the progressive left-hemisphere lateralization of functions throughout the life-span.

Of principal importance in the present context is the view of Goldberg and Costa (1981) that the right cerebral hemisphere is particularly geared to the handling of tasks involving *inter*modal integration, whereas the left cerebral hemisphere is particularly adept at *intra*modal processing. Among the implications of this position is the notion that right-hemisphere systems are particularly necessary for dealing with novel information processing demands for which the individual has no preexisting code, whereas systems within the left cerebral hemisphere are seen as particularly adept at the handling, elaboration, and stereotypic application of codes or descriptive systems (such as natural language) that have already been learned. (According to Goldberg and Costa, a descriptive system implies any set of discrete units of encoding or rules of transformation that can be successfully applied to the processing of a certain class of stimuli.)

In this view, it is the right hemisphere that is crucial for dealing with situations in which no task-relevant descriptive system is immediately available in the person's cognitive repertoire. Such situations can be of at least two types: (1) orientation in a novel task when no descriptive system is immediately apparent, but the task is ultimately recognized as relevant to an existing one and (2) orientation in a novel task to which none of the available descriptive systems can be successfully applied. In both cases, left-hemisphere systems are expected to take a leading role in the routinized, stereotypic application of any particular descriptive system, once it has been "assembled" for use by right-hemisphere systems. In situations of the first type just described, the role of the right hemisphere would be particularly salient only for the initial orientation period, whereas, in type 2 situations, right-hemisphere systems would be particularly active during both initial orientation and during the assembling of the new descriptive system. Thus, a right-to-left shift of relative hemispheral control over cognitive processes is thought to take place as these processes undergo functional transformation in the course of their development.

EXAMPLES OF RIGHT- AND LEFT-HEMISPHERE DIFFERENCES AND INTERACTIONS

Normal Reading

An example from the development of the learning-to-read process illustrates how some of these dimensions of right- and left-hemisphere differences apply. For the sake of discussion, the learning-to-read process is divided into three stages.

Stage 1

Initially, by definition, reading is a novel task. Although the child has an existing descriptive system (i.e., natural language), this system has not yet been related to print. In consequence, one would expect an initial emphasis of right-hemisphere systems in orientation to the reading task.

Stage 2

Even as initial orientation subsides and the task of relating graphic characters to the preexisting though still immature natural language system become of prime concern, it would be expected that the right hemisphere would be quite actively engaged in "assembling" the units of print (e.g., graphemes) for linkage with the units of the preexisting linguistic system (e.g., phonemes). The necessity for the active exploration of the shapes and contours of letters, syllables, words, and phrases would be expected to involve right-hemisphere systems in direct proportion to the *novelty* of these various print units. Thus, one would envision the right hemisphere being particularly involved in the initial phases of letter-by-letter, syllable-by-syllable, word-by-word, and phrase-by-phrase analyses. The intervals between each of these initial learning phases (i.e., the consolidation of learning "plateau" phases) would be expected to invoke a more salient contribution by left-hemisphere systems, since these are thought to be more concerned with the utilization of routinized descriptive systems. That is, the extent to which letters, syllables, words, and phrases become "routines" would specify the extent of the increased involvement of left-hemisphere systems, with reciprocal deemphasis on right-hemisphere systems. The final levels of letter, syllable, word, and phrase reading, insofar as only speed of reading is concerned, would invoke, almost exclusively, left-hemisphere systems, if the process is to be efficient. The left hemisphere's facility with automatization and fixation on a single mode of representation and execution would be particularly suited for this. At the level of automatization, then, the reading process would be expected to invoke primarily left-hemisphere systems.

Stage 3

Finally, there is the dimension of reading comprehension. On the assumption that the most efficient way to do two things at once is to automatize one so as to enable concentration on the other, it would seem reasonable to suppose that the most efficient method of analyzing, organizing, and synthesizing (i.e., comprehending) text would be to have the left-hemisphere processes automatized, thus "freeing" one to concentrate on and emphasize the functioning of right-hemisphere systems and their unique role in dealing with novelty, informational complexity, and intermodal integration (i.e., achieving new meanings from the text). In these ways, one can envision the relative salience of the right and left cerebral hemisphere systems changing in predictable ways as a function of levels of competence in the various stages of the learning-to-read process. The similarities evident between this particular view and that of Bakker (1979) are very clear and are intended.

Two Subtypes of Learning Disabilities

The preceding description of the learning-to-read process illustrates the application of this model to the normal acquisition of a cognitive skill. The following serves as an illustration of how the model can be used to explain some relevant neuropsychological dimensions in children who exhibit two different types of learning disability: (1) extreme deficiency in rapid reading and reading comprehension (group R-S) and (2) well-developed rapid reading, less well-developed reading comprehension, and outstandingly poor mechanical arithmetic (group A).

In a number of related studies reviewed in Chapter 2 (Rourke & Finlayson, 1978; Rourke & Strang, 1978; Strang & Rourke, 1983), differences in the neuropsychological profiles of two groups of learning-disabled children (groups R-S and A) have been highlighted. Both of these groups are constituted on the basis of their patterns of academic performance. Group R-S exhibits extremely poor performance in reading (word recognition) and spelling and somewhat better, though still clearly impaired, levels of performance in mechanical arithmetic. Group A exhibits extremely well-developed word-recognition and spelling skills, but outstandingly poor performance in mechanical arithmetic.

In terms of the model under consideration, group R-S exhibits the type of performance that would be expected were these children to be suffering from deficiencies in left-hemisphere systems, whereas group A exhibits a pattern that would be expected from those experiencing deficiencies in systems subserved primarily by the right hemisphere. The following descriptions of the ability profiles of these two groups of children illustrate these points. In addition, attempts are made to employ aspects of these findings to speak to issues raised within the model with respect to both the normal and abnormal ontogenetic development of cognitive skills.

Group A

Group A children usually exhibit very clear strengths in areas that require rote verbal learning; regular phoneme–grapheme matching skills (e.g., virtually all of their misspellings are of the phonetically accurate variety); amount of verbal output; and verbal classification in terms of regular categories such as color, size, and genus. They also exhibit fairly normal simple, stereotyped motor movements (e.g., finger tapping) and simple tactile-perceptual abilities. However, these children tend to be quite deficient in skills such as visual-spatial organization and synthesis, fine psychomotor coordination under speeded-up conditions, some fine tactile-perceptual abilities, and higher-order concept-formation and problem-solving abilities. The tactile-perceptual and psychomotor deficits are usually more marked on the left side of the body. Although they are able to read words rapidly, their reading comprehension scores are much lower than are their word-recognition scores. This deficiency in reading comprehension appears to be related to their very poor concept-formation and problem-solving abilities, as reflected in their extremely deficient performance on the more difficult aspects of the Halstead Category Test and on a number of other tasks of a nonverbal problem-solving nature that require the utilization of feedback in a flexible fashion in problem-solving situations (see Chapter 2 and Rourke, Bakker, Fisk, & Strang, 1983). Another feature of their performance that serves to limit their comprehension is their tendency to process print in a rigid, programatic fashion, possibly reflecting a penchant for excessive routinization of performance. Indeed, the outstanding feature of their performance in mechanical arithmetic, aside from the obvious visual–spatial deficiencies in evidence, is their failure to orient themselves in an appropriate fashion to the changing requirements of successive arithmetic problems and to comprehend and/or utilize in a systematic fashion those rules that are necessary for complex aspects of arithmetic calculation (see Chapter 2).

In terms of the model under consideration, group A children seem to have acquired the automatization of reading through an essentially "isolated" set of left-hemisphere systems. The basis for their problems in other types of learning and adaptation appears to be that they have very deficient right-hemisphere systems or limited access to them, thus rendering the processing and integration of novel stimuli and ideas very difficult and sometimes impossible. Indeed, such children typically experience difficulty even in the understanding of facial expressions of emotion; their social relationships tend to be routinized and stereotyped; and the quality of their affect and speech tends to be "flat" and stereotyped. These modes of relating, together with their virtual inability to deal with complex visual-spatial arrays, especially in novel or otherwise stressful situations, would suggest that the functions of orientation, intermodal integration, and synthesis—postulated to be the "province" of right-hemisphere systems in this model—are all but inoperative, or at least inaccessible.

Even the typical oral language of such children reflects a lack of input from right-hemisphere systems. For example, their expressive speech could be best characterized as being of the "cocktail party" variety, containing much verbiage but little if any conceptual content. Indeed, they are often said by speech pathologists to be suffering from a content disorder of speech and/or to be deficient in the pragmatic aspects of language.

More generally, their capacity for verbal classification, especially in terms of standard, simple categories, far exceeds their ability to understand simple conservation tasks. This is particularly noteworthy, since progressive levels of conservation are thought to be necessary for facility in classification, at least according to Piaget (1954). If we assume that such abilities are primarily a reflection of the adequate functioning of right-hemisphere systems and that verbal classification in a standard, systematic fashion is primarily mediated by the left hemisphere, and if we assume additionally that the normal course of ontogenetic development involves a progression from the salience of right-hemisphere systems to the salience of left-hemisphere systems, one would have to conclude that group A children have essentially "skipped over" at least some of the ordinary prerequisites (i.e., some aspects of right-hemisphere development) for this dimension of cognitive development. In a sense, they seem to have proceeded to the utilization of left-hemisphere systems for these adaptational purposes. In fact, the excessive automatization, stereotypic behavior, and perseveration noted in their behavior would seem to reflect precisely the state of affairs to be expected were left-hemisphere systems to be functioning in a virtually independent fashion.

A summary of the representative predictions for group A children that can be derived from this model, and empirical findings and conclusions, where available, are presented in the following list. These are meant to serve merely as illustrations of the heuristic value of the model, to demonstrate the extent to which deductions from it serve to reinforce confidence in its basic elements, and to provide some notion of how empirical findings can serve to enhance its articulation and development.

1. *Prediction*: Group A children should have difficulty in the initial phases of reading, because orientation to and intermodal integration of the novel aspects of print are important at this stage in the learning-to-read process.

Finding and conclusion: It is the case that these children have problems in the initial phases of reading acquisition. However, by the time they have achieved levels of performance in visual-spatial abilities approximately equivalent to those of a 6- to 7-year old (which generally occurs when they are approximately 9 to 10 years of age), these difficulties are no longer noticeable. This would suggest that the feature-detection requirements for accurate rapid reading (word recognition) do not exceed the ordinary competencies of the 6- to 7-year old.

2. *Prediction*: Eventually, group A children should not experience difficulties with rapid reading.
Finding: They become very adept at rapid reading.

3. *Prediction*: These children should have some difficulties in reading comprehension. Although word reading becomes automatized as a result of the operation of intact left-hemisphere systems, the analysis of novel ideas as well as formulations relating to the content, organization, and synthesis of concepts are hampered by dysfunctional and / or inaccessible right-hemisphere systems.
Finding and conclusion: Typically group A children become much more adept at word recognition and rapid reading than at reading comprehension. More generally, they seem to learn little from experience of any sort, rarely modifying their behavior in response to those situations that would be expected to involve "new information" of a conceptual kind for children of their age. It appears as though their capacity for simultaneous accounting and assessing of the various components of any novel problem situation, such as that posed by complex meaningful text, is extremely limited.

Group R-S

The situation with respect to the R-S group is almost exactly the reverse of that seen in group A. Children in group R-S exhibit many poor psycholinguistic skills (especially those that tax the acoustic-verbal system) and some limited facility with the more rote and overlearned aspects of verbal skills, within a context of extremely well-developed visual-spatial analysis, organization, and synthesis abilities. They are free of fine tactile-perceptual deficiencies, except in the case of dysgraphesthesia, where the symbolic aspects of the stimuli probably constitute the principal limitations with respect to their performance. They exhibit good psychomotor coordination, and their nonverbal problem-solving and concept-formation skills are excellent. Typically, they deal extremely well with novel circumstances; that is, they analyze the situation, organize the elements of stimulus arrays, deal systematically and flexibly with competing problem-solving strategies, benefit from informational feedback, and adapt flexibly to changing circumstances. In terms of the model under consideration, children in this group appear to have extremely well-developed right-hemisphere systems.

The deficiencies exhibited by the R-S group are primarily those thought to be subserved by left-hemisphere systems. These children tend to speak very little; their speech and language are rather immature and impoverished; and they often fail to understand much more than simple auditory-verbal assertions, especially if these are delivered rapidly and are nonredundant, not elaborated with nonverbal cues, not delivered distinctly, and not repeated. Their reading is slow and labored; they may read no more than simple sight-words, and their misspellings are often characterized by phonetic inaccuracy. To say the least, they appear not to have developed automatized verbal skills to any considerable extent.

A summary of illustrative predictions, findings, and conclusions for group R-S children is provided in the following list. Once again, the purpose of this exercise is to provide some notion of the empirical side of this theory-building enterprise.

1. *Prediction*: Group R-S children should have less difficulty in the early stages of reading when using the "look–say" method, if the "say" dimension is provided.

Finding: Reading drills involving the provision of simultaneous visual and auditory input are usually successful with such children, at the time of training; however, this new learning soon extinguishes. After a short time, when only the graphic elements of words are presented, they are able to provide sounds for only very simple, usually one-syllable sight-words.

2. *Prediction*: Group R-S children should have no facility with rapid reading.

Finding: These children do not read rapidly; rather, their reading is slow, syllable-by-syllable, and labored.

3. *Prediction*: These children should have marked difficulty in reading comprehension at an age-appropriate level because their slow, labored approach to the decoding of individual words places an enormous load on their memory capacities. The amount of interference occasioned by the absence of any facility in rapid reading would be expected to preclude the efficient storage of meaningful units in short-term (working) memory and, hence, in long-term (semantic–procedural) memory.

Finding: These children exhibit very poor reading comprehension.

4. *Prediction*: These children should exhibit enhanced comprehension when meaningful material of age-appropriate difficulty is presented orally, at an average rate of speed, and with appropriate inflections and prosody. This should help to circumvent some of the mnestic problems occasioned by their protracted nonroutinized word-decoding attempts, wherein little if anything in the way of syntactical, prosodic, and other essentially nonverbal cues is available for use.

Finding: These children give evidence of much better comprehension under these conditions than when required to read the same material on their own.

5. *Prediction*: Group R-S children should be aided somewhat in reading comprehension by giving them the context of the phrases, sentences, and paragraphs that they are attempting to read, and by presenting the material at a normal rate of speed.

Finding and conclusion: Older children of this type often comprehend the meaning of phrases, sentences, and paragraphs fairly well, in spite of the fact that they cannot read many of the words in them. It appears as though they are able, under these and other types of cuing and pacing conditions, to "fill in" the conceptual gaps occasioned by their limited word-recognition skills.

The differences evident in the performances of groups R-S and A can be accounted for reasonably well in terms of the Rourke (1982) model, especially with respect to differences in the dimensions of novelty versus stereotypy and content versus execution. Together with these dimensions, there are additional aspects of this model that would seem appropriate for the explanation of other empirical findings in the area of children's learning disabilities, as discussed in Chapter 2. One of these is spelling disability. The aspects of the model that are of particular interest in this connection are those having to do with the left hemisphere's hypothesized facility for dealing with unimodal processing and intramodal integration. However, before delving into the applications of these dimensions to the understanding of spelling disabilities, an explanation of some of their possible information-processing ramifications is necessary.

Goldberg and Costa (1981) maintain that "the left hemispheral advantage appears to be twofold: (1) processing of elemental units of the linguistic signal (probably secondary to a more basic acoustic and/or oral-motor advantage); and (2) processing of those aspects of the linguistic signal and/or code which are based upon fixed systems of rules, and manipulations of the code or internal derivations within the code according to these rules" (p. 160).

Their first point stresses the specialized unimodal processing carried out by the left hemisphere, and the specialization of left-hemisphere systems for the integration of information processing within a particular mode or elemental unit. Point 2 emphasizes the proclivity of these elemental units to function in a fixed and stereotyped fashion in terms of their own inner dynamics. Both of these attributed emphases, if accurate, would suggest that the left hemisphere should have different systems—reasonably separated, if not isolated from each other—that are capable of functioning rather independently (i.e., in terms of their own rules and without recourse to activity in other systems). In addition, the advantage of the left hemisphere for the processing of the acoustic aspects of the linguistic signal is emphasized. Taking these particular aspects of left-hemisphere superiority into consideration, we can attempt to apply them to some of the data that have been generated in our studies of children who exhibit severe problems in spelling.

Subtypes of Spelling Disability

We have shown that 9- to 14-year-old disabled spellers who are equated for impaired level of performance in spelling, but who differ markedly with respect to levels of phonetic accuracy in their misspellings, are also quite different with respect to their performance on a variety of linguistic tasks (Sweeney & Rourke, 1978). The phonetically accurate (PA) disabled spellers perform at superior levels to phonetically inaccurate (PI) disabled spellers on all psycholinguistic skills except for those that require the successive activities of decoding word strings and encoding word strings in reply to them. The superiority of the PA spellers is also evident in reading or word recognition. At the same time, PA spellers are inferior to normal spellers (who do not differ from PAs with respect to the level of phonetic accuracy of their misspellings) on a wide variety of psycholinguistic skills, including reading or word recognition.

Thus, although the ability of PA disabled spellers to hear phonemes would seem to be at least as well developed as is that of normal spellers, their capacity to match these phonemes with appropriate graphemes for the activity of spelling is quite deficient. This would suggest, in turn, that the PA speller's "phonetic analyzer"—to use Luria's term (presumably, the secondary region of the left temporal lobe)—is intact, but that there is some degree of functional disorganization of the temporo-parieto-occipital region (the tertiary area) of the left hemisphere, which interferes with the more complex levels of phoneme–grapheme analysis and synthesis. This would lend support to the Goldberg and Costa (1981) contention that the left hemisphere has a penchant for the processing of elemental units of the linguistic signal (in this case, phonemes). Further-more, the "normal" capacity of the PA spellers to process phonemes in terms of a fixed system of rules and to manipulate the code according to these rules (i.e., to spell in a phonetically regular fashion) would highlight the specialized unimodal processing of which the left hemisphere is capable, its emphasis upon integration within a particular mode or elemental unit, and the proclivity of its elemental units to function in a stereotyped fashion in terms of their own inner dynamics.

These same points would apply to group A children and to other types of hyperlexics. It will be recalled that group A children become excellent spellers and that their misspellings are virtually all of the phonetically accurate variety. Their penchant for sameness, lack of no-velty, and the routine unfolding of behavior in an almost robotlike fashion would suggest that even relatively well-functioning secondary and tertiary zones within the left hemisphere will still eventuate in rigid adherence to inflexible routines in the elaboration of a descriptive system when (as is hypothesized in this case) right-hemisphere systems are dys-functional or inaccessible.

What may be taken as a corollary of the tendency for the left hemisphere to specialize in unimodal systems and intramodal integra-tion, with a corresponding penchant for the stereotyped elaboration of unidimensional codes, is that one would expect statistical clustering algorithms to isolate distinct subtypes of individuals on the basis of those information-processing abilities and deficits that are thought to be sub-served primarily by the left hemisphere. This would be particularly the case for algorithms that stress the patterning of abilities such as the Q-type of (inverted) factor analysis. Another example from the results of our own investigations should serve to illustrate this point.

Empirically Derived Reading Disability Subtypes

Through the application of the Q-type factor analysis, we isolated three reliable subtypes of disabled readers at the age level of 7 to 8 years

(Petrauskas & Rourke, 1979). All of these children exhibited deficiencies in psycholinguistic skills, but to varying degrees. These three subtypes were characterized by patterns of neuropsychological abilities and deficits that were hypothesized to be reflective of dysfunction maximally involving the temporal (subtype 1), temporo-parietal (subtype 2), and frontal (subtype 3) regions of the left cerebral hemisphere (Petrauskas & Rourke, 1979; Rourke & Strang, 1983).

It is particularly interesting to note in this connection that Goldberg and Costa (1981), when discussing the left hemisphere's relatively strong predisposition for elemental phonetic processing, point to the particular importance of the temporal planum, parietal operculum, and pars opercularis of inferior frontal gyrus, which correspond precisely with the hypothesized areas of maximal dysfunction of the Petrauskas and Rourke (1979) subtypes 1, 2, and 3, respectively. It is also interesting to note that approximately 20% of the disabled readers in the Petrauskas and Rourke study were less reliably classified and 30% were not classified at all. This "unexplained variance" may be a reflection of disordered brain function within more than one left-hemisphere system; right-hemispheral dysfunction; or other, nonbrain-related causes for disabled reading. However, a close examination of the controls exercised in this study would suggest that the latter is quite unlikely, and the results also would suggest that the first two account for very little of the unexplained variance. What is clear is that the three subtypes that were identified fit quite precisely with the features of left-hemisphere anatomical and behavioral specialization outlined by Goldberg and Costa (1981) and that more than 90% of the normal readers included in this study did not load in these reading-disabled subtypes.

Group A Arithmetic and Social Learning Disabilities

A final consideration within this model is the interrelated dimensions of social perception, socioemotional adaptation, and "personality." All of these aspects of the child's functioning have two features in common: They are influenced heavily by learning and they seem to be particularly sensitive to early developmental experiences. Once again, on both counts, aspects of the Goldberg and Costa (1981) model, which were incorporated within the Rourke (1982) model, provide us with a convenient structure within which to explain our research findings.

If children are to develop normally, from a socioemotional point of view, it would seem quite necessary for them to benefit from experiences, especially with their human environment. The skill development resulting therefrom would be expected to contribute to the process of social adaptation, a notion that plays a central role in virtually every theory of personality development. As outlined in Chapters 2 and 3, the capacity to benefit from new learning situations, especially those emerging during early developmental stages, has been the focus of much of our recent work regarding group A learning-disabled children. These children exhibit patterns of neuropsychological abilities and deficits that are strongly suggestive of relatively dysfunctional right-hemisphere systems. Of particular interest is the cause-and-effect relationship that seems to obtain between their pattern of neuropsychological abilities and deficits and their problems in arithmetic and in socioemotional adaptation (Rourke, 1982; Rourke & Fisk, 1981). Examining some features of their performance in both of these areas will serve to illustrate this point. (For more examples, see Chapter 2.)

Arithmetic

A qualitative analysis of the arithmetic errors of group A children reveals that they attempt calculations for which they have little understanding. Although there is a tendency for children in group A to misread mathematical signs, probably as a result of confusion with respect to the visual-spatial characteristics of the signs, it appears that the most pervasive of their limitations in arithmetic involves an impoverished understanding of mathematical concepts. For instance, in the case of subtraction questions involving several steps, it is sometimes found that such children end up with an answer that is something in excess of the minuend, even though some numbers have been subtracted. This kind of difficulty would suggest at least a limitation in the child's ability to check the adequacy of the solution.

An important aspect of the model under consideration is that the limits of the arithmetic performance of group A children are viewed as related directly to their pattern of neuropsychological abilities and deficits. Visual-spatial and visual-perceptual deficiencies such as those exhibited by these children can contribute to problems in reading similar-looking calculation signs, forming numbers, aligning columns of numbers, attending to all numbers in the operation, observing directionality, carrying out procedures in a systematic fashion, and generally organizing the work. The psychomotor deficiencies characteristic of these children (e.g., problems with motor steadiness in the kinetic disposition) can also contribute directly to many of the mechanical arithmetic difficulties that they exhibit.

A plausible explanation of these problems requires consideration of the children's neuropsychological deficiencies within a developmental framework. As outlined earlier, these neuropsychological deficiencies include visual spatial and visual-perceptual problems, bilateral psychomotor deficiencies, and bilateral tactile-perceptual difficulties. It would seem probable that these difficulties have been present since birth and that they were more exacerbated at that time for most, if not all, such children. If this be the case, it would stand to reason that these deficiencies—within a context of adequate auditory-perceptual and, eventually verbal expressive capacities—would alter substantially the normal course of development of sensorimotor skills for these children. This, in turn, might contribute to considerable developmental deviation in the acquisition of cognitive skills. In fact, many theorists (e.g., Piaget, 1954) consider the adequacy of sensorimotor experience, particularly in the first 2 years of life, to be an important determinant of the child's potential for later concept-formation abilities.

The suspected inability of group A children to generate and deal with elementary, age-appropriate nonverbal concepts as well as their problems in establishing cause-and-effect relationships on a physical, concrete basis during infancy and early childhood (supposedly one of the principal intellectual achievements of the first 2 years of life) may, in turn, have limited their ability to develop more abstract levels of thought. This would seem to have rather direct implications for the learning of mathematics, since the understanding of even rather simple mathematical operations requires some degree of nonverbal abstract conceptualization.

The concept-formation and problem-solving difficulties that these children experience with mathematics also appear to extend into other realms of their academic development and everyday life. School subjects that involve logical nonverbal reasoning abilities (e.g., many aspects of natural science) prove to be quite difficult for them, unless lessons are taught in a step-by-step fashion that encourages rote learning. Furthermore, as already pointed out, reading comprehension capacities are almost always much less developed than are word-analysis skills in such children.

Socioemotional Adaptation

With respect to the dimensions of socioemotional adaptation, it should be pointed out that it is common to find that group A children have interactional problems with their peers, often becoming rather withdrawn in novel social situations or appearing to be somewhat "out of place." One factor possibly contributing to this situation is their somewhat deficient (nonverbal) logical reasoning abilities, particularly under novel conditions (Strang & Rourke, 1983). New social situations seem to pose a serious problem for them because of the large number of cues that must be interpreted properly in order to understand fully the social interactions that are proceeding and the specific requirements demanded from or for each individual in them. Another factor that seems to contribute to their social inadequacies is their difficulty in attending to and/or providing nonverbal cues. Facial expressions, hand movements, body postures, and other physical gestures are forms of nonverbal communication that are important for success in novel social situations. As noted in Chapter 3, we have shown that the perception and understanding of these forms of communication seem to be deficient in such youngsters (Ozols & Rourke, 1985). Furthermore, their overutilization of programatic, routinized language in social situations tends eventually to alienate those persons with whom they are interacting. Trite phrases are often utilized in an almost perseverative fashion, suggesting that these children do not fully appreciate the novel, changing aspects of even ordinary social intercourse. Their inflexibility, overuse of routinized linguistic and nonverbal performance patterns, and failure to appreciate the consequences of their behavior render smooth adaptation to social situations virtually impossible.

Summary

The foregoing observations and generalizations, which are drawn principally from our empirical studies of such children, should be sufficient to illustrate the point under consideration, namely that group A children exhibit deficiencies in intermodal integration, problem solving, and concept formation (especially in novel situations), and that they have a profound inability to benefit from experiences that do not fit or mesh well with their existing, overlearned descriptive system (i.e., natural language). In a word, with respect to the model under consideration, they exhibit what may be referred to as quite deficient right-hemisphere capacities within a context of well-developed, modality-specific, intramodal, routinized, and stereotyped left-hemisphere skills.

PREDICTIONS OF LATERALIZED CEREBRAL ACTIVATION

Before summarizing and concluding our discussion of this model, brief mention should be made of the sorts of predictions regarding patterns of cerebral activation, for both normal and disabled learners, that can be deduced from it.

First, in visual half-field studies and in dichotic listening studies, children and adults should exhibit a left-visual-field and a left-ear "superiority," respectively, for material that is relatively unfamiliar and/or not typically handled in a routine, programatic fashion. Examples include music for the nonmusician, as well as most emotional stimuli. This should occur if responses to novelty and the extraction of meaning are roles for which the right hemisphere is particularly suited and, presumably, activated.

In a similar vein, to the extent that the analysis of print remains a novel and/or nonprogramatic task (as is the case for the 12-year-old disabled reader), the right hemisphere may be more than normally activated under EEG-evoked potential "challenges" that involve words. For the poor reader, it may be the case that both left- and right-hemisphere systems are partially activated by words, whereas in the normal 12-year-old reader the print is handled routinely (principally by the systems within the left hemisphere) while the right hemisphere is "freed" for intermodal processing (i.e., the extraction of meaning). Thus, print that involves lengthy scrutiny before any novel and meaningful content is possible would be expected to eventuate in much left-hemisphere activation and very little right-hemisphere activation. Only by raising the novel, meaningful content of the prose would one expect to find a situation obtaining in the good reader that is similar to that in the disabled reader (i.e., evidence of equal activation of both hemispheres or more activation of the right than of the left cerebral hemisphere).

These predictions should serve to illustrate this model's potential for encompassing aspects of behavior that have only quite recently been subjected to close neuropsychological scrutiny, and which hold considerable promise with respect to our understanding of the various dimensions and stages of information processing for both normal and disabled learners.

CONCLUSION

This finishes our discussion of the Rourke (1982) model. As mentioned at the outset of this chapter, almost all of the foregoing has been cast in very similar terms to the manner in which this model first appeared. This was done so that the reader might appreciate the historical context of the development of the model, especially with regard to the research and theory formulation that followed it.

Before proceeding to a description of the NLD syndrome and model, it might be well to mention the work of other investigators who have subsequently arrived at conclusions and formulations regarding group A subjects that bear a more than passing similarity to those outlined in the 1982 model and the reports that have been emanating from our laboratory since the early 1970s. These would include the work of Tranel, Hall, Olson, and Tranel (1987), with regard to right-hemisphere developmental learning disability; Voeller (1986), with regard to right-hemisphere deficit syndrome; and Weintraub and Mesulam (1983), with regard to developmental learning disabilities of the right hemisphere. All of these investigators report findings on group A children that are largely consistent with those reported in this book up to this point. It is, of course, reassuring that such replications have been carried out in laboratories other than our own; however, of more crucial importance are the validation studies of this learning-disability subtype, which have been reviewed recently by Fletcher (1985).

CHAPTER FIVE

The NLD Syndrome: Characteristics, Dynamics, and Manifestations

The foregoing chapters have outlined the research results and the rather limited theoretical formulations relating to differences between right- and left-hemisphere systems, which have led to the characterization of group A and other subtypes of learning-disabled youngsters. The current chapter focuses on the manifestations of the group A learning-disabled subtype in persons with "developmental" presentations of the syndrome and in those with well-documented neurological disease, disorder, and dysfunction. Hereafter, I will refer to the set of characteristics that were isolated in the group A child, in addition to a number of other dimensions outlined herein, as the "NLD syndrome." The emphasis is on explaining the interactions within and between the sets of neuropsychological abilities and deficits that are thought to be operative in the NLD syndrome, and the neurophysiological elements and interactions that are inferred to give rise to the NLD syndrome in its various manifestations.

We begin with a description of the characteristics of the NLD syndrome and then move to a brief explication of the dynamic interactions among and between the various levels of this syndrome's basic and derived manifestations. We turn then to a more specific discussion of these dynamics. This is followed by a listing of the types of neurological disease, disorder, and dysfunction of childhood and adolescence, wherein its characteristics are particularly evident. The effort will be to answer the following questions regarding the NLD syndrome:

- What are its characteristics?
- How do these characteristics interact?
- Who exhibits the syndrome?

All of this is to prepare the ground for dealing with a discussion of the NLD model in Chapter 6.

SUMMARY OF CHARACTERISTICS

In this outline of the characteristics of the NLD syndrome, a clear, although minimally articulated, description of each of the dimensions (assets and deficits) in question is provided. To these are added statements regarding the developmental course of each. Within each major category, some notions regarding hypothesized interactional dynamics within and between categories are mentioned. These dynamics are expanded upon later in the chapter, where the interactions of these characteristics are discussed in detail.

Two features of this description of NLD syndrome characteristics should be borne in mind:

1. Because of our focus on children and adolescents, manifestations of NLD in persons within these developmental stages are emphasized.
2. This description is couched in terms of the "developmental" manifestation of the NLD syndrome, that is, in terms of its characteristics in a child who has been so afflicted since her or his earliest developmental stages. Some modifications in the manifestations of the syndrome are necessary when we turn to considerations of the onset of the syndrome in an older child, adolescent, or adult who has enjoyed a normal early developmental course.

Note on Dynamics. The following summary of the assets and deficits of the NLD syndrome should be viewed within a specific context of cause and effect relationships; that is, the basic neuropsychological assets and deficits are thought to lead to the secondary neuropsychological assets and deficits, and so on, within the four categories of neuropsychological dimensions. Moreover, these assets and deficits are seen as causative vis-à-vis the academic and socioemotional/adaptive aspects of the syndrome. In this sense, the latter dimensions are, essentially, dependent *variables (i.e., effects rather than causes) in the NLD syndrome. Figure 5.1, provided later, may be of some assistance in understanding the dynamics that are proposed to obtain in the NLD model.*

Neuropsychological Assets

Primary Assets

Simple motor. Simple, repetitive motoric skills are generally intact, especially at older age levels (middle childhood and beyond).

Auditory perception. After a very early developmental period when such skills appear to be lagging, auditory perceptual capacities become very well developed.

Rote material. Repetition and/or constancy of stimulus input—especially through the auditory modality, but not confined to it—is well appreciated. Repetitious motoric acts, including some aspects of speech and well-practiced skills such as handwriting, eventually develop to average or above-average levels.

Secondary Assets

Attention. Deployment of selective and sustained attention for simple, repetitive verbal material (especially that delivered through the auditory modality) becomes very well developed.

Tertiary Assets

Memory. Rote verbal memory and memory for material that is readily coded in a rote verbal fashion becomes extremely well developed.

Verbal Assets

Speech and language. Following an early developmental period when linguistic skills appear to be lagging, a number of such skills emerge and develop in a rapid fashion. Excellent phonemic hearing, segmentation, blending, and repetition and very well-developed receptive language skills and rote verbal capacities are evident, as are a large store of rote verbal material and verbal associations, and a very high volume of speech output. All of these characteristics tend to become more prominent with advancing years.

Academic Assets

Following initial problems with the visual–motor aspects of writing and much practice with a writing instrument, graphomotor skills (for words) reach good to excellent levels. Following initial problems with the development of the visual–spatial feature analysis skills necessary for reading, good to excellent single-word reading (decoding) skills are in evidence. Single-word spelling-to-dictation skills also develop to above-average levels. Misspellings are almost exclusively of the phonetically accurate variety. Verbatim memory for oral and written verbal material can be outstanding in the middle to late elementary school years and thereafter.

Neuropsychological Deficits

Primary Deficits

Tactile perception. Bilateral tactile-perceptual deficits are evident, usually more marked on the left side of the body. These deficits tend to become less prominent with advancing years.

Visual perception. There is impaired discrimination and recognition of visual detail and visual relationships, as well as outstanding deficiencies in visual-spatial-organizational abilities. Deficits in this area tend to increase with advancing years.

Complex psychomotor. Bilateral psychomotor coordination deficiencies are prominent; these are often more marked on the left side of the body. These deficits, except for well-practiced skills such as handwriting, tend to increase in severity with age.

Novel material. As long as stimulus configurations remain novel, they are dealt with very poorly and inappropriately. Difficulties in age-appropriate accommodation to, and a marked tendency toward overassimilation of, novel events increase with advancing years.

Secondary Deficits

Attention. Attention to tactile and visual input is poor. Deficiencies in visual attention tend to increase over the course of development, except for material that is programatic and overlearned (e.g., printed text). Deployment of selective and sustained attention is much better for simple, repetitive verbal material (especially that delivered through the auditory modality) than for complex, novel nonverbal material (especially that delivered through the visual or haptic modalities). The disparity between attentional deployment capacities for these two sets of materials tends to increase with age.

Exploratory behavior. There is little physical exploration of any kind. This is the case even for objects that are immediately within reach and could be explored through visual or tactile means. A tendency toward sedentary and physically limited modes of functioning increases with age.

Tertiary Deficits

Memory. Memory for tactile and visual input is poor. Deficiencies in these areas tend to increase over the course of development, except for material that is programatic and overlearned (e.g., spoken natural language). Memory for nonverbal material, whether presented through the auditory, visual, or tactile modalities, is poor if such material is not readily coded in a verbal fashion. Relatively poor memory for complex, meaningful, and/or novel verbal and nonverbal material is typical. Differences between good to excellent memory for rote material and impaired memory for complex material and/or that which is not readily coded in a verbal fashion tend to increase with age.

Concept formation, problem solving, strategy generation, and hypothesis testing; appreciation of informational feedback. Marked deficits in all of these areas are apparent, especially when the concept to be formed, the problem to be solved, and/or the problem-solving milieu are novel or complex. Also evident are significant difficulties in dealing with cause-and-effect relationships and marked deficiencies in the appreciation of incongruities (e.g., age-appropriate sensitivity to humor). Most noticeable as formal operational thought becomes a developmental demand (i.e., in late childhood and early adolescence), deficits in these areas tend to increase markedly with advancing years, as does the gap between performance on rote (overlearned) and novel tasks.

Verbal Deficits

Speech and language. Mildly deficient oral-motor praxis, little or no speech prosody, and much verbosity of a repetitive, straightforward, rote nature are characteristic. When paraphasic errors are in evidence, these are much more likely to be of the phonological than of the semantic variety. Also typical are content disorders of language, characterized by very poor psycholinguistic pragmatics (e.g., "cocktail party" speech) and reliance upon language as a principal means for social relating, information gathering, and relief from anxiety. All of these characteristics, except for oral-motor praxis difficulties, tend to become more prominent with advancing years.

Academic Deficits

Graphomotor. In the early school years, there is much difficulty with printing and cursive script; with much practice, handwriting most often becomes quite good.

Reading comprehension. Reading comprehension is much poorer than is single-word reading (decoding). Deficits in reading comprehension, especially for novel material, tend to increase with advancing years.

Mechanical arithmetic and mathematics. There are outstanding relative deficiencies in mechanical arithmetic as compared to proficiencies in reading (word-recognition) and spelling. With advancing years, the gap between good-to-excellent single-word reading and spelling and deficient mechanical arithmetic performance widens. Absolute level of mechanical arithmetic performance only rarely exceeds the Grade 5 level; mathematical reasoning, as opposed to programatic arithmetic calculation, remains poorly developed.

Science. Persistent difficulties in academic subjects involving problem solving and complex concept formation (e.g., physics) are prominent. The gap between deficiencies in this type of complex academic endeavor and other, more rote, programatic academic pursuits widens with age.

Socioemotional/Adaptational Deficits

Adaptation in novel situations. There is extreme difficulty in adapting to (i.e., countenancing, organizing, analyzing, and synthesizing) novel and otherwise complex situations. An overreliance on prosaic, rote (and, in consequence, inappropriate) behaviors in such situations is common. These characteristics tend to become more prominent with advancing years.

Social competence. Significant deficits are apparent in social perception, social judgment, and social interaction skills; these deficits become more prominent as age increases. There is a marked tendency toward social withdrawal and even social isolation with advancing years.

Emotional disturbance. Often characterized during early childhood as afflicted with some type of acting-out or conduct disorder, such children are very much at risk for the development of "internalized" forms of psychopathology. Indications of excessive anxiety, depression, and associated internalized forms of socioemotional disturbance tend to increase with advancing years.

Activity level. Children who exhibit the syndrome are frequently perceived as hyperactive during early childhood. With advancing years, they tend to become normoactive and eventually hypoactive.

SUMMARY OF DYNAMICS

The principles relating to the dynamics that are inferred to be operative between the various levels and dimensions of the NLD model are presented schematically in Figure 5.1, while the assets and deficits that comprise the NLD syndrome are summarized in Table 5.1. More specific explications of these principles are contained within the next section of this chapter.

DETAILS OF CHARACTERISTICS AND DYNAMICS

This section is designed to provide a fuller description of the characteristics of the NLD syndrome and to place them within the context of their developmental dynamics. It is structured in a manner that assumes that the reader will make reference to Table 5.1 and Figure 5.1 whenever necessary to follow the discussion.

Note on Terminology. In all of what follows in this section, I refer to the "developmental presentation" of the NLD syndrome, by which I mean the presentation that appears to have been evident at birth or shortly thereafter, and which is not complicated by subsequent neurological disease, disorder, or dysfunction. Although the same general principles—and especially the dynamics of the syndrome—hold for other children and adolescents who have experienced a normal course of development before suffering an untoward event (e.g., significant craniocerebral trauma) that eventuates in the NLD syndrome, there are important differences between the "developmental" and "other" presentations of the syndrome, the latter being due to neurological disease superimposed upon a normally developing brain. These differences are especially evident when we compare the neuropsychological presentations of children whose early months and years of cognitive development have been "normal" with those of children who

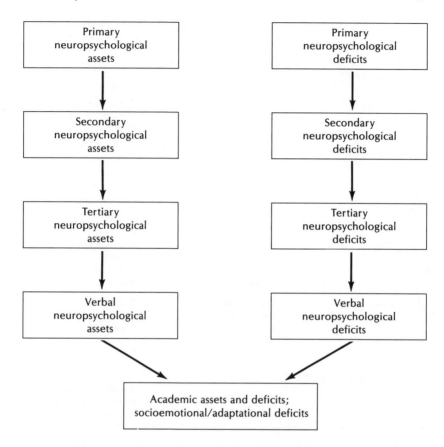

FIGURE 5.1. Key dynamic relationships among categories of assets and deficits, according to the NLD model.

have been affected adversely by the elements and dynamics of the NLD syndrome since a very early developmental stage.

Neuropsychological Assets and Deficits

Early Presentation: Primary Neuropsychological Skills and Abilities

The principal neuropsychological asset of children who exhibit the NLD syndrome is their capacity to deal with information delivered through the auditory modality. Virtually all other assets of such children appear to

TABLE 5.1. Summary of NLD Assets and Deficits

	Assets	Deficits
Neuropsychological		
Primary	Auditory perception	Tactile perception
	Simple motor	Visual perception
	Rote material	Complex psychomotor
		Novel material
Secondary	Attention (auditory; verbal)	Attention (tactile; visual)
		Exploratory behavior
Tertiary	Memory (auditory; verbal)	Memory (tactile; visual)
		Concept formation
		Problem solving
Verbal	Phonology	Oral-motor praxis
	Verbal reception	Prosody
	Verbal repetition	Phonology > semantics
	Verbal storage	Content
	Verbal associations	Pragmatics
	Verbal output (volume)	Function
Academic	Graphomotor (late)	Graphomotor (early)
	Word decoding	Reading comprehension
	Spelling	Mechanical arithmetic
	Verbatim memory	Mathematics
		Science
Socioemotional/adaptational	???	Adaptation to novelty
		Social competence
		Emotional stability
		Activity level

flow from this basic strength. It should be pointed out, however, that in infancy it is often suspected that children who are eventually shown to have a developmental presentation of the NLD syndrome are "hard of hearing." This impression is reinforced by a discernible delay in the acquisition of speech. (Fortunately, advances in evoked audiometry now make it possible to discern the integrity of the auditory apparatus at very tender ages.) Adding to the seriousness of this situation during the first months and years of these children's lives is the fact that developmental milestones, including speech, are clearly delayed. Indeed, it is fairly common for such children to be scrutinized carefully during their early months of life, with the differential diagnostic possibilities of mental retardation, deafness, and/or severe (pervasive) emotional disturbance in mind.

This being the case, it should come as no surprise that parents and other caretakers are overjoyed when such children utter their first sounds of speech. This joy mounts thereafter as the children progress through the various stages of speech and language development at what seems to be an above-normal rate of speed. This is usually accompanied by the parents' selective and effusive positive reinforcement of this linguistic output, with a correlative disregard for the fact that the children are still not making normal progress in the attainment of other developmental milestones, especially those having to do with locomotor and manipulative skills. These children remain essentially sedentary, exploring the world not through vision or locomotion, but rather through receiving verbal answers to questions posed about the immediate environment. An example of the differences between the style of behavior exhibited by normally developing children and those with NLD may serve to illustrate the serious shortcomings in terms of cognitive development that the early limitations of the NLD syndrome entail.

Consider what a normal child entering toddlerhood would do in a sitting room filled with antiques and other visually interesting objects. The following scenario may very well ensue, once her parent is distracted: She spots a visually interesting vase on a table across the room from where she is sitting. She gets to her feet and toddles over to the table, feels the vase for a moment, picks it up, and then tosses it in the air. As the vase crashes to the ground, she hears her parent shriek, "My God! That's Aunt Gertrude's vase!" This is followed quickly by a swat across the child's nether portions and subsequent admonitions to avoid Aunt Gertrude's vase (and all other like it) in the future. Contrast this scenario with that which is likely to ensue when a child with NLD is involved in the same situation: Lounging with his parent in the sitting room, he sees the vase but makes no move to wend his way over to it. Rather, he asks his parent what it is. The reply comes immediately: "That's Aunt Gertrude's vase." He pays no further heed to the vase. Instead, he proceeds to ask more questions about objects in the room, and his parent responds with verbal information about them.

Let us consider what each of these children learns in this process. The "normal" child spots the interesting object, then mobilizes her locomotor resources to reach it. While so doing, she maintains her path to the object by periodically sighting it, and, when first encountering the object, she touches it. This is followed by lifting it and tossing it in the air and by the sounds of the object crashing to the floor, the rattle of its scattered bits to the four corners of the room, and her parent's plaintive cry. This is followed quickly by a feeling of pain and further verbal utterances by the parent. It is quite possible that this sequence of events has occasioned the following: elementary, though crucial, notions regarding means–ends relationships and the sense of efficacy and confidence that mobilizing one's resources successfully to accomplish the end (examine the target object) can promote; the notion that the object remains constant in the face of perturbations of the retinal size of the light reflecting from it; the realization that the object has a smooth surface and that it has a mass that allows her to lift it; some elementary notions of the interactions between aerodynamics and gravity as the object flies through the air; the realization that an object that is smooth and of this weight disintegrates when it encounters a relatively immovable object such as a wooden floor; the name of the object; the consequences of engaging in this type of activity; and further verbal labels and qualifiers for this activity and for the object involved therein.

In all of this, it should be noted that, for the normal child, the object was assigned a label (name) only *after* many of its physical features had been encountered, if not explored, in some detail. I would submit that, for the child in late infancy and early toddlerhood, this is not only the most *common* manner in which many labels are assigned to objects, but also the *preferred* manner for this naming activity to transpire at this time. The prerequisites for this sequence of events, of course, are the neuropsychological dimensions of tactile and visual perception, complex psychomotor skills, and the capacity to deal with novelty. Deficits in all of these are thought to constitute the basis of the NLD syndrome.

Thus, when we turn to a consideration of the learning that has transpired for the NLD child regarding Aunt Gertrude's vase, we are presented with a very simple answer to our query, namely, that he has probably learned that the object is a "vase" and that it bears some relationship to "Aunt Gertrude." Nothing else.

Even within the context of this simple example at a relatively tender age, we can see the beginnings of the complex interactions that tend to transpire between and among the neuropsychological abilities and deficits of children with NLD. For example, it would appear quite likely that such children will become progressively less likely to engage in physical exploration of their environment, precisely because the patent auditory channel and its rapidly emerging receptive linguistic correlates provide information without the difficulties and large expenditures of energy attendant upon the engaging of deficient psychomotor skills for such purposes. Indeed, the more often and the more elaborate the parents' and other caretakers' verbal answers to these children's questions, the more likely it becomes that they will engage in sedentary rather than exploratory behaviors. This, in turn, reduces the opportunities for encountering truly novel stimuli, with consequent negative repercussions for an already diminished capacity to deal with such stimuli. In all of this, of course, it is clear that the reinforcement histories of such children would be expected to exacerbate or partially mollify some of these effects.

As a final consideration with respect to early presentations of basic neuropsychological skills and abilities, some note should be made regarding simple motor skills. It is a basic principle of the NLD syndrome and model that the reduction of novelty to familiarity and the invocation of the stereotypy that comes from sustained practice of simple motoric acts should lead to proficiency in them. Thus, it should come as no surprise that, throughout this developmental process, particular skills such as graphomotor activities, although extremely difficult for the child initially, tend to be mastered to a considerable extent as a result of extensive practice. This mastery is a function of the repetitive nature of the task and the familiar nature of the surroundings within which it is to be executed.

Attention, Exploratory Behavior, and Memory

The patent auditory channel of the NLD child, in concert with difficulties in dealing with visual and tactile signals, would be expected to increase the likelihood of good auditory attentional deployment and poor tactile and visual attentional deployment. In addition, it would be expected that, for the distance senses (audition and vision), the gap between "attention" within these modalities would tend to widen with advancing years.

Tactile perception is a special case: Little effort is required to engage this sensory modality; it can be developed within the proximate space of even a virtually immobile child; it can be "practiced" extensively by a child who is prone to engage in repetitive, rote behavior. For all of these reasons, it is expected that NLD children will eventually show little or no marked, "hard," signs of deficiencies in the tactile modality, including the capacity to deploy attention within this modality. Hence, although visual attention (and other skills and abilities that are dependent upon this rather basic processing level) would be expected to decline relative to age-appropriate norms, such would not be expected in the case of the "contact" sense of touch.

Exploratory behavior is expected to be quite deficient in terms of frequency and quality because of (1) the NLD child's penchant for rote material, (2) a correlative avoidance of novelty (because of an inability to "handle" its informational processing demands), (3) problems in deploying complex psychomotor skills (e.g., climbing), and (4) a tendency to prefer the auditory over the visual modality for the processing of information. All of these features should conspire early in the child's life to limit exploration of the environment; thus, for example, it is expected that the child will come to prefer to *hear* about the environment rather than to *see* or to *touch* it.

It is a small step from the latter developmental point to expectations regarding relative proficiency in auditory (especially auditory-verbal) memory over visual memory. It should come as no surprise that several investigators have found that the auditory-verbal memory skills of group A children are superior to their visual memory skills (e.g., Fletcher, 1985). Similar results have been obtained recently in our own laboratory (Brandys, Rourke, & Shore, 1989). The chain of events in the case of the child exhibiting NLD would seem to suggest very strongly that well-developed attention and memory for auditory stimuli and poorly developed attention and memory for visual stimuli follow a cause-and-effect sequence as follows: good or poor sensory-perceptual capacity→good or poor attentional deployment skills→good or poor memory. Furthermore, the interactions along this sequence are important; that is, it would be expected that, just as all biological organisms have a strong tendency to practice what they do well and to avoid what they do poorly, the very existence of a "strength" (auditory analysis) would be expected to interfere with the practice of a "weakness." In other words, within the perception→attention→memory sequence, it would appear quite probable that the rich will get richer and the poor, poorer. It is only with a balance between and among these capacities that one would expect "normal" information processing development to occur.

Concept Formation, Problem Solving, Strategy Generation, Hypothesis Testing, and Appreciation of Informational Feedback

The analysis, organization, and synthesis of information constitute the cognitive building blocks that lie at the basis of the ability to form and modify concepts, generate reasonable solutions to complex problems, apply these solutions in a testable fashion, and deal systematically with feedback regarding the acceptability of solutions to the problems. Another important basis for such activity is the capacity to tolerate and even relish novelty.

It should be remembered that classic studies of creative thinking (e.g., Hutchinson, 1949a, 1949b) have, without exception, pointed to the necessity of knowing (i.e., studying, examining, exploring, and remembering) all feasible aspects of the problem to be solved, if a creative solution is to be the outcome. Although Edison may have been off the mark somewhat in his estimates of the relative contributions of perspiration (99%) and inspiration (1%) to creativity, there is no doubt that the former is a prerequisite for the latter. And, it is in the former activities that NLD children are not prone to engage. Such engagement would require systematic, careful visual (and sometimes) tactile exploration of the evidence; perhaps complex psychomotor manipulation of the elements of the problem; a capacity for dealing with novel material; and memory for what one has seen during the exploration of the problem. These capacities are deficient in NLD children and, in the developmental presentation of this syndrome, would be expected to have been deficient since their earliest days.

Previous references to Piaget's notions regarding the genesis of intelligent behavior are certainly relevant here. The "contributions" of the sensorimotor phase of development for the eventual attainment of formal operational thought are necessary to the series of events just proposed. The disabilities in concept formation and other forms of higher cognitive processes that are exhibited by NLD children are seen as a fairly direct consequence of a failure to acquire these cognitive building blocks.

Speech and Language

In this formulation of the NLD syndrome, it is hypothesized that NLD children's speech and language assets are fairly direct reflections of their more basic neuropsychological assets, and that deficits in this area are similarly a reflection of more basic neuropsychological deficits.

Well-developed capacities for auditory perception, attention, and memory would seem to be excellent (and virtually sufficient) for the development of natural language in nonretarded persons who attain some even rather elementary enunciatory and word-finding skills. Thus, good phonemic hearing, segmentation, and blending capacities should lead to good-to-excellent verbal reception, verbal repetition, verbal storage, and verbal associative skills. These are characteristics of NLD children that tend to develop to above-average, even extreme, degrees; such developments are accompanied by increasingly larger volumes of verbal output.

In these children's early years, oral-motor praxis problems are in evidence, though rarely severe or even moderate in degree. But, mild difficulties in the enunciation of complex, multisyllabic words tend to persist throughout development. These are inferred to be one reflection of a more general problem in praxis that persists over time.

More telling deficits evident in the linguistic performance of NLD children include their problems in appropriate prosody and, more important, the sometimes grossly deficient content and pragmatics of their linguistic productions. The deficiencies in content and pragmatics are viewed as direct results of difficulties in concept formation and other higher-order cognitive skills. These in turn are inferred to be reflections of more basic neuropsychological deficiencies, as is the marked tendency to favor the phonological aspects of oral communication over its semantic content.

The end result of this pattern of linguistic deficits is poor "functional" language, a concept that is conveyed somewhat by the aforementioned deficiencies in linguistic pragmatics. It is included here because the means–ends relationships that language promotes in normal persons are notably absent from the spoken and written language of NLD persons. This shortcoming is usually evident as a general and pervasive deficit touching virtually every aspect of their communicative behavior. It almost always appears to reflect a much more basic problem in appreciating the functional role that language can play in achieving one's goals.

Academic Assets and Deficits

After a rather slow start in kindergarten, Grade 1, and perhaps into Grade 2, NLD children exhibit remarkable gains in single-word reading (decoding). It is not uncommon for such children to be rated on word decoding at the Grade 6 level when they are in Grade 3, at the Grade 9 level when they are in Grade 4, and at the Grade 11 level when they are in Grade 5. Indeed, beyond Grade 3, their word-recognition skills are usually well in excess of their age-expected grade level.

An obvious question to pose at this juncture is, Why are children who exhibit the NLD syndrome often thought to be "at risk" for reading disability when they are in kindergarten and Grade 1? The answer is quite straightforward. Although something of an oversimplification, there are two prerequisites for beginning reading: (1) the natural language capacity (language age) of a 5½- to 6-year-old and (2) the visual-spatial feature-analysis skills of the average child of this age. In the case of NLD children, the first prerequisite is usually attained by the chronological age of 4 years; however, the latter may not occur until they are almost 7. Once this is attained, the rapid development of their word-decoding skills becomes quite apparent and begins to match or even exceed their apparent language age.

It is quite common to find that even very experienced kindergarten teachers and school psychologists are convinced that their NLD students are at risk for reading failure upon entry to kindergarten. This "diagnosis" is usually confirmed after several months of experience with the child. Most often, remedial techniques are applied to such children, in an effort to enhance their reading-readiness skills. When they do, in fact, begin to read single words and then virtually skyrocket in this skill, there is the sense among their caretakers that this good to excellent performance in reading is a result of their interventions. Unfortunately for their egos, the same result would have occurred if they had virtually ignored the child—or tried yoga, or megavitamin therapy, or any other currently "hot" intervention technique that enjoys little or no empirical support for its efficacy. The fact of the matter is that NLD children will read at least well, and probably at a superior level, regardless of what is done to help them. All they need to accomplish this is access to print and a marginally supportive educational milieu. (More examples of such assumed—and unfounded—therapeutic "efficacy" for the NLD child will be outlined in subsequent sections of this book.)

The spelling ability of NLD children follows a course similar to that exhibited in single-word reading; however, there is an added complication. In written spelling, rather than oral spelling, it is necessary to engage in graphomotor activity. Of course, this involves basic neuropsychological deficits exhibited by NLD children in the areas of tactile-perceptual, visual-perceptual, and complex psychomotor skills. As already noted, NLD children's graphomotor skills are usually very poor during the primary grades of school. Often, such poor script—which is produced quite slowly and laboriously—is difficult for teachers and even for the children themselves to decipher. This situation would be expected to lead to an underestimate of the children's capacities in spelling during the early elementary school years. Once again, however, with the advent of the visual–spatial prerequisites noted earlier in connection with single-word reading, spelling performance begins to pick up. Smooth, coordinated handwriting may be seen as early as Grade 5 or 6, but in any case it will develop at some point.

It should be emphasized that graphomotor script becomes smooth and effortless even though it involves the most basic neuropsychological deficits included within this syndrome. This would appear to attest to the capacity of NLD children to routinize this activity completely. As noted in connection with the Rourke (1982) model, the capacity for such routinization and stereotypic application is thought to be a process for which left-hemisphere systems are particularly geared.

Another important dimension of NLD children's spelling performance is its fidelity to the phonetic composition of the words to be spelled. This is certainly a predictable attribute, in view of these children's basic neuropsychological assets in phonemic hearing, segmentation, and blending. Misspellings are almost exclusively of the phonetically accurate variety (e.g., "nacher" for nature; "okupie" for occupy). In fact, it is common to find that better than 95% of their misspelled syllables are rendered in a phonetically accurate manner. (See Sweeney & Rourke, 1978, for an explanation of our syllable-by-syllable system for assessing phonetic accuracy.) This rather high percentage becomes more than an idle curiosity when we see it in light of the fact that English is approximately 75% "regular" with respect to phoneme–grapheme correspondences. (This should be compared with virtually 100% phoneme–grapheme correspondences in Finnish.) It is also the case that normal adolescent and adult misspellings tend to be approximately 75% phonetically accurate. Taking these facts together, it becomes clear that English-speaking NLD children and adolescents are "hyperphonetic" in the analysis of words to be spelled.

Other aspects of this tendency to accentuate the phonetic qualities of words (often to the detriment of their semantic content) can be seen in NLD children's tendency to make far more phonological than semantic paraphasic errors during sentence repetition tasks. It is as though, when given the opportunity to "choose" between the way words sound and what they mean, the former triumphs over the latter.

Mechanical arithmetic poses considerable difficulty for these children. As pointed out in Chapters 2 and 4 in connection with the arithmetic performance of group A children, the problems in evidence appear to reflect basic neuropsychological deficits in visual-spatial-organizational and psychomotor skills, appreciation for novel data, and the interrelated dimensions of concept formation, strategy generation, and hypothesis testing. Limitations in judgment and reasoning tend to predominate in the productions of older NLD children; these would include their apparent failure to realize the inappropriateness of answers to arithmetic problems. Perseveration and failure to shift set in serial arithmetic problem solving would appear to reflect such difficulties, as do the related penchants for stereotyped, routinized, programatic unfolding of behavior in any number of situations.

Rarely does the mechanical arithmetic prowess of NLD adolescents or adults exceed the Grade 5 to 6 level. Up until the Grade 2, 3, or even 4 level, it is sometimes not possible to see the emerging discrepancy between word-recognition and spelling (high) and arithmetic (low), because of the nature of the arithmetic problems that are considered to be within the ken of the 7- to 8-year-old child. After this point and beyond, however, this discrepancy is easily discernible.

One particular proclivity of NLD children and adolescents in mechanical arithmetic deserves further comment because it bears upon subsequent discussions regarding frankly brain-damaged individuals. This is their marked tendency to "forget to remember." This phrase applies to individuals who have stored memories that would be applicable to a given situation but who fail to realize that a particular time and place call for the particular stored material in question. Thus, it can usually be shown that 10-year-old NLD children "know" how to "carry" and "borrow" but do not access these stored arithmetic rules when it would be appropriate to do so. This problem is easy to understand when we consider that normal people do not ordinarily commit to memory the *occasions* when particular memories need to be employed, but rather "trust" that their judgment at any particular time will be such that a decision to scan memory for the appropriate rule will be forthcoming. Note that this "trust" is probably a long-term consequence of the repeated assurances that ensue from efficacious problem-solving in novel situations.

This interaction between memory/remembering and good and poor higher-order reasoning skills is analogous to the difference between skilled and unskilled mathematicians. The skilled mathematician would never dream of committing, say, the Pythagorean theorem to memory, but would instead "reason it through" when required to do so. Those who must commit the theorem to memory so as to regurgitate it when asked to do so are to be applauded for their verbal memory and the capacity to respond appropriately to the cue that calls forth this remembered material. What they may very well lack is the capacity to engage in elementary mathematical thinking. In this connection, it is often found that NLD adolescents perform much better in secondary school mathematics courses than they did in elementary school arithmetic. This is so to the extent that the secondary school mathematics courses require verbatim memory for theorems, corollaries, and the like, as opposed to adaptive problem solving. When NLD adolescents turn to subjects such as physics, their difficulties in concept formation, problem solving, and hypothesis testing become very apparent. These deficiencies are compounded by their failure to benefit from informational feedback in such problem-solving situations.

Socioemotional/Adaptational Deficits

As with the academic deficits just described, the socioemotional difficulties of NLD children appear to result from interactions among and between their neuropsychological assets and deficits. The following are some examples of such interactions:

1. Deficits in social judgment would appear to result from more basic problems in reasoning, concept formation, and the like, which also lie at the root of difficulties in mechanical arithmetic and scientific reasoning.

2. Difficulties in visual-spatial-organizational skills are reflected in problems in identifying and recognizing faces, expressions of emotion, and other subtle nonverbal identifiers of important dimensions of human communication.

3. Lack of prosody, in conjunction with a high volume of verbal output, tends to encourage negative feedback from those who find themselves forced to listen to the seemingly endless recitation of dull, drab, colorless statements that these youngsters seem impelled to deliver. In a word, the type of speech and the language characteristics exhibited by such children tend to alienate them from others, thus increasing the probability that they will experience socioemotional/adaptational difficulties.

4. The tactile-perceptual and psychomotor prowess required for smooth affectional encounters, in conjunction with NLD children's typically inappropriate judgments regarding nonverbal cues, renders intimate encounters all but impossible.

5. Adaptability to novel interpersonal situations is the hallmark of socially appropriate individuals. The combination of aversion to novelty,

failure sometimes even to appreciate that an event is in fact novel, and poor problem-solving and hypothesis-testing skills conspires to render spontaneous, smooth adaptation to the constantly changing milieux of social groups and the interactions nascent therein all but impossible for NLD individuals.

The dynamics of the changes in activity level that are quite commonly seen in the developmental presentation of the NLD syndrome are relevant within this context. Typically, NLD children are seen as hyperactive when they are 4 or 5 years of age. They are constantly getting in the way of others, they seem to be disinhibited, they bump into other persons and objects, and they persist in such behavior over protracted periods of time. These manifestations of the sensorimotor and other deficiencies of the NLD syndrome are often taken as indicators of the presence of hyperactivity and, presumably, an underlying attention deficit disorder as well. For this reason, methylphenidate is often prescribed for such youngsters. After a time in school, their behavior tends to "normalize" in terms of activity level, and they may no longer be medicated. Thereafter (usually during the middle of the elementary school years), it is noticed that they appear to be somewhat hypoactive.

This is, of course, another example of a situation wherein it would be easy to infer that the pharmacological agent and/or any other form of intervention employed (e.g., behavioral shaping) has been effective in the reduction of hyperactivity. The fact that the child reads and spells well after a course of such therapy also suggests that any underlying attentional deficit has also been "cured."

It must be pointed out, however, that the natural history of these children involves moving from apparent hyperactivity through normoactive behavior and then on to a hypoactive response style. This occurs largely, if not exclusively, as a result of the rebuffs and outright physical punishments that NLD children experience as a result of their failure to anticipate the consequences of their actions. Agemates and adult caretakers tend to react very negatively to such shenanigans. And, since there is no reason to think that NLD children are anhedonic, there is good reason to infer that the negative consequences of their behavior will eventuate in the reduction of activity level. Of course, a very unfortunate by-product of this reduction in activity level is an even further reduction in exploratory behavior, with the negative consequences that this can entail for the children's cognitive development.

These few examples should suffice to illustrate the main point of this discussion, namely, that socioemotional/adaptational deficiencies are, essentially, dependent variables in the NLD matrix. As with academic deficits, they arise out of a common mix of neuropsychological abilities and deficits that all but insures that they will occur and grow in intensity with the passing of years. Unfortunately, the eventual social and personal outcome for those with NLD is almost never a pleasant one. Withdrawal, isolation, and loneliness are common. Some of the more dire consequences of this combination of events are dealt with in Chapter 7.

EMPIRICAL TEST OF THE DEVELOPMENTAL DYNAMICS OF THE SYNDROME

The discussion of the characteristics and dynamics of the NLD syndrome up to this point has contained a mixture of empirical findings and many statements and generalizations of an essentially clinical nature. It would be well to introduce some data now that address the developmental dynamics of the NLD syndrome in a rather more direct, empirical fashion.

One issue that arises within the context of research on the NLD syndrome is whether and to what extent its manifestations may change over the course of development. Evidence that such changes do occur was presented by Rourke, Young, et al. (1986). In that study, we demonstrated that adults who exhibit the NLD syndrome were much more deficient (relative to age-based norms) than were their younger NLD counterparts (relative to their age-based norms) on tests for psychomotor coordination, problem solving, and concept formation. The two groups performed at similar levels, relative to age-based norms, on tests for linguistic functioning. It was also possible to infer that socioemotional disturbance was more marked in the NLD adults than in the NLD children who were studied. However, the adult sample was obviously biased in this regard, since it was made up of individuals who had been referred for neuropsychological assessment from a hospital-based psychiatry service.

In an attempt to deal with the implications of the NLD model vis-à-vis these suggestions, it would be instructive to examine the results of other, more recent exploratory investigations carried out in our laboratory. These studies should also serve to illustrate rather more generally how deductions from the NLD model may be subjected to empirical test. The studies in question (Casey & Rourke, 1989; Rourke & Casey, 1989) involved attempts to expand the previously reported (Rourke, Young, et al., 1986) initial observations of apparent age-related changes in the presentation of the NLD syndrome in adults, to include the determination of the presence of such changes within the 7- to 15-year-old age range.

Subjects were selected for study in accordance with the neuropsychological, academic, and socioemotional criteria of the NLD syndrome. These subjects were divided into two groups on the basis of age: a "young" group (7 to 8 years of age) and an "old" group (9 to 15 years of age). Based on the NLD model and previous research, it was expected that the older NLD subjects would exhibit (1) relative stability (i.e., age-appropriate advances) in rote verbal skills, word recognition, spelling, and simple motor skills; (2) relative declines in visual-spatial-organizational skills, mechanical arithmetic, and complex psychomotor skills; and (3) increased severity of psychopathology, especially of the internalized variety, and a decrease in hyperactivity.

Hypotheses

The specific hypotheses of the study were as follows:

Hypothesis 1. It was expected that (a) WISC VIQ and PPVT IQ would not differ between older and younger children, (b) PIQ for younger children would exceed that of older children, and (c) the difference between WISC VIQ and PIQ (favoring VIQ) would be larger for older than for younger children.

Hypothesis 2. It was expected that (a) WRAT Reading and Spelling standard scores would be higher for older than for younger children, (b) WRAT Arithmetic standard scores would be higher for younger than for older children, and (c) the difference between WRAT Reading and Spelling on the one hand and WRAT Arithmetic on the other (favoring WRAT Reading and Spelling scores) would be larger for older than for younger children.

Hypothesis 3. It was expected that, the more complex and novel the motor or psychomotor task, (a) the poorer would be the performance of both groups relative to age-based norms and (b) the poorer would be the age-corrected performance of the older children as compared to the younger ones. The hierarchical order of simplicity versus complexity and rote versus novel is as follows: Grip Strength, Finger Tapping Speed, Holes Test, Foot Tapping Speed, Mazes Test, Grooved Pegboard Test. (Name-writing speed does not fit well within this hierarchy. It was assumed that name writing would be a well-practiced task for older but not for younger children; hence, it was expected that it would be carried out better, relative to age-based norms, by the older than by the younger children.) (See Rourke, Fisk, & Strang, 1986, for a description of the measures involved in the testing of this hypothesis.)

Hypothesis 4. It was expected that (a) all NLD children would perform below normal limits on the Underlining Test and (b) the younger children would perform better (relative to age-based norms) than would the older children on the 14 subtests of the Underlining Test. (The Underlining Test is timed, it has rather novel task requirements, and some of its subtests appear to require fairly complex visual-spatial-organizational skills for successful performance. See Rourke, Fisk, & Strang, 1986, for a description of the test.)

Hypothesis 5. It was expected that the following would obtain on the scales of the Personality Inventory for Children (PIC): (a) more concern regarding academic achievement and the need for "intellectual screening" among the older as compared to the younger children; (b) significant elevations on the Adjustment scale and on those scales that contribute to the internalized psychopathology factor (Depression, Withdrawal, Anxiety, Psychosis, Social Skills) would be in evidence for both age groups; (c) moderate but significant elevations of the F ("degree of concern") scale, and higher F scales for the older children; (d) higher scores on scales that contribute to the internalized psychopathology factor for the older than for the younger children; and (e) elevations on the Hyperactivity scale would be higher for the younger than for the older children.

Subject Selection and Characteristics

Twenty-nine subjects who fit the criteria for the NLD syndrome (with the exceptions noted shortly) were chosen from a large sample of children who had undergone neuropsychological assessment for a variety of reasons. Most of the children in this sample had been referred for neuropsychological assessment because they were manifesting some type of learning disability for which it was thought that brain impairment might be a contributing factor; two had well-documented brain lesions. Each of the features of the syndrome was evident in each of the test protocols examined. Exceptions to this rule were the applicability of criteria relating to nonverbal problem solving and concept formation for the younger children, and criteria relating to difficulty in adapting to novel or otherwise complex situations for all children. In the latter case, it was not always possible to determine precisely that the child was experiencing such difficulties. Aspects relating to socioemotional functioning were not considered in the formation of the groups.

The subjects were between the ages of 7 years, 0 months and 15 years, 0 months of age at the time of testing. Twenty-one of them had undergone neuropsychological assessment only once; seven had been tested twice; one was tested three times. Since this study was exploratory in nature, all 38 testings of all subjects were included in these analyses. The test protocols of these subjects were divided into those at the younger age level (7 years, 0 months to 8 years, 11 months) and those at the older age level (9 years, 0 months to 15 years, 0 months) at the time of the test. There were 7 sets of test results at the younger age level and 31 sets of test results at the older age level. WISC Full Scale IQs ranged from 64 to 105; all subjects obtained a WISC Verbal IQ of at least 88. There were 14 girls' and 15 boys' sets of protocols examined in the study.

Measures

The following measures were employed: VIQ, PIQ, and 11 (excluding Mazes) subtests from the WISC (Wechsler, 1949); the Reading, Spelling, and Arithmetic subtests from the Wide Range Achievement Test (WRAT; Jastak & Jastak, 1965); IQ from the Peabody Picture Vocabulary Test (PPVT; Dunn, 1965); Finger Tapping Test and Name Writing Speed (Reitan & Davison, 1974); Foot Tapping, Holes, Mazes, and Grooved Pegboard Tests from the Klove–Matthews Motor Steadiness Battery (Klove, 1963); the 1 control and 13 critical subtests of the Underlining Test (Rourke & Gates, 1980); and the Validity, Adjustment, Academic Achievement, Intellectual Screening, and 8 clinical scales of the PIC (Wirt et al., 1977). All tests were administered in a standardized manner by technicians trained extensively in the administration of these tests to children referred for neuropsychological assessment.

Results

Table 5.2 contains the means and standard deviations for age, WISC and
PPVT IQ scores, and WRAT subtest scaled scores. The following analysis shows how these figures apply to each of the hypotheses set forth for
this study.

*Note on Findings. In view of the exploratory and essentially heuristic aims
of this study, the relating of its results does not include reference to the
statistical significance of those differences for which it was possible to conduct appropriate statistical tests. Rather, the results are couched in terms of
trends and other features that serve to enhance their heuristic purposes.*

Hypothesis 1. The results of this investigation revealed the following: (a) VIQs for the younger and older subjects were virtually identical;
(b) PIQs for older subjects were lower than for younger subjects;
(c) VIQ–PIQ discrepancies (favoring VIQ) for the older subjects were
larger than those for younger subjects; (d) there were four WISC Verbal
subtest scaled scores higher and two lower for the older versus younger
subjects; (e) all five of the WISC Performance subtest scaled scores were
lower for the older versus younger subjects; and (f) PPVT IQs for the
older subjects were higher than those for the younger subjects. These six
sets of results coincided with the expectations of hypothesis 1.

TABLE 5.2. Means (Standard Deviations) for Age; WISC VIQ, PIQ, and FSIQ;
PPVT IQ; and WRAT Reading, Spelling, and Arithmetic Scores

	Test protocols			
	Younger children ($n = 7$)		Older children ($n = 26$)	
Age (years)	8.1	(0.54)	11.7	(1.8)
WISC				
VIQ	104.9	(6.1)	100.1	(10.2)
PIQ	88.1	(7.8)	78.4	(10.7)
FSIQ	96.7	(7.6)	88.8	(10.7)
PPVT IQ	106.4	(7.7)	107.2	(8.1)
WRAT standard score				
Reading	110.1	(9.0)	115.7	(6.3)
Spelling	103.6	(9.1)	108.2	(5.7)
Arithmetic	91.9	(7.0)	83.3	(10.6)

Hypothesis 2. The following results were obtained: (a) WRAT Reading and Spelling scores for older subjects were higher than were those for younger subjects; (b) the Arithmetic scores for older subjects were lower than those for younger subjects; (c) the difference between Reading and Spelling (high) and Arithmetic (low) was larger for older than for younger subjects. These three sets of results were in accord with the predictions of hypothesis 2.

Hypothesis 3. The following results, all couched with reference to appropriate age-based norms for the tests in question, were germane to this hypothesis: (a) grip strength was about the same for the older versus younger subjects, and all scores were within or above normal limits; (b) finger-tapping scores for the older subjects were poorer than for the younger subjects; (c) all four scores for both groups were within normal limits on the Holes Test, and three of the four scores for the older subjects were superior to those for the younger subjects; (d) there were virtually no differences between younger and older subjects in foot-tapping scores, and all of these scores were well below normal limits and poorer (relative to age-based norms) for both age groups than were scores on finger-tapping; (e) all scores for the Mazes Test for the younger subjects were superior to those of the older subjects; (f) Grooved Pegboard scores for both hands for the younger subjects were mildly impaired, those for the older subjects were markedly impaired, and the discrepancy between the scores of the younger and older subjects was more marked on this complex psychomotor task than on any of the other motor and psychomotor tasks; (g) name-writing time scores for the nondominant hand for the younger subjects were significantly impaired, dominant-hand scores for both groups were normal and virtually indistinguishable, and nondominant-hand scores for the older subjects were within normal limits and superior to those of the younger subjects.

Hypothesis 3(a) was partially confirmed, since the hierarchy of actual performance for the two groups combined was in the following order, from best to worst (hypothesized order from 1 through 6 is in parentheses): Grip Strength (1), Holes Test (3), Mazes Test (5), Finger Tapping Speed (2), Foot Tapping Speed (4), Grooved Pegboard Test (6). For the most part, hypothesis 3(b) was also upheld: It was quite clear that, in general, the more complex and novel the motor or psychomotor task (e.g., Mazes and Grooved Pegboard Tests), the more marked was the discrepancy between older and younger subjects, favoring the performance of the latter. Also, name-writing speed of the older subjects (nondominant hand) was superior to that of the younger subjects.

Hypothesis 4. The following results were of interest in this connection: (a) with the exception of the younger subjects' performance on one subtest (#11), the levels of performance on the Underlining Test fell below normal limits; and (b) in 10 of 14 instances, the performance of the younger subjects was superior to that of the older subjects. The expectation regarding superior performance of the younger subjects was upheld.

Hypothesis 5. With respect to the PIC scores, the following should be noted: (a) the F ("degree of concern") scale for the older subjects was somewhat higher than that for the younger subjects; (b) concern over academic achievement and the need for intellectual screening were higher in the older versus younger subjects, and elevation on the Intellectual Screening scale was within the pathological range for the older subjects; (c) elevations on eight of the nine clinical scales (excluding Somatic Concern) were higher for the older than for the younger subjects; (d) elevation on the Hyperactivity scale was somewhat higher for the older versus younger subjects; and (e) elevations on Development, Depression, Delinquency, Withdrawal, Anxiety, Psychosis, and Social Skills scales were higher for the older versus younger subjects. With the exception of the Delinquency scale, these elevations are those most typically seen in children who exhibit internalized forms of psychopathology. With only very minor exceptions, the predictions embedded within hypothesis 5 were confirmed.

Discussion

Hypothesis 1. All of the expectations contained within hypothesis 1 were upheld. These results were in line with the notion that the rote, overlearned skills tapped by the WISC VIQ subtests and the PPVT are those at which NLD children are expected to become increasingly adept with the passing of time. On the other hand, NLD children are expected to have increasing difficulties with the more novel, timed problem-solving tasks that make up the bulk of the task demands of the WISC Performance subtests.

Hypothesis 2. For the same reasons just enunciated, the overlearned skills of single-word reading and spelling would be expected to improve at rates exceeding those expected on the basis of age alone. This is expected to be accompanied by a decline in age-appropriate advances in the more complex problem-solving skills that are involved in mechanical arithmetic. The novelty of the particular arithmetic tasks included on the WRAT Arithmetic subtest, the essentially changing nature of the task demands of successive questions on this subtest, and the timed nature of the task all would be expected to put the NLD child at an increasing disadvantage with advancing age. Thus, it is expected that NLD children will practice behaviors and skills that call for the exercise of their assets (e.g., in rote verbal skills), at the expense of those that require expertise in their areas of deficit (e.g., in novel problem solving).

Hypothesis 3. This hypothesis was largely confirmed. There were virtually no differences between the groups on the more simple motor skills tapped by the Grip Strength and Holes Tests. However, marked differences were in evidence between the groups on the more complex psychomotor skills tapped by the Mazes and, especially, the Grooved Pegboard Tests. In the latter instances, the differences between the groups were very evidently in favor of the younger subjects. These differences on the more complex psychomotor tasks are reminiscent of those evident in the studies of Rourke and Telegdy (1971) and Rourke, Dietrich, and Young (1973). From a different and more pertinent perspective for the current study, these differences were especially similar to those noted in the Rourke, Young, et al. (1986) investigation.

More generally, with advancing years, it would appear that NLD children show no particular difficulties with rote tasks, whether these are verbal in nature (hypothesis 1), academic in nature and involving essentially programatic verbal skills (hypothesis 2), or straightforward motor skills with little complex sensory-perceptual analysis and integration required. On the other hand, NLD children exhibit increasing difficulties on tasks that require visual-spatial-organizational skills, involve complex problem solving, and demand the coordination of several sources of sensory-perceptual information for their successful completion. All of these predictions are entirely in accord with the principal tenets of the NLD syndrome.

Hypothesis 4. This hypothesis was strongly supported. The explanations for this support are those just mentioned.

Hypothesis 5. With advancing years, it is clear that the indications of psychopathology generally, and internalized socioemotional disturbance particularly, increase in NLD children. It is not clear that advances in age are accompanied by a lessening of hyperactivity.

Summary

Strong support was offered by this study for predictions based on the hypothesized dynamics of the NLD syndrome. Further work in this area should involve strictly cross-sectional and, especially, strictly longitudinal studies of NLD children. The results of this exploratory study would suggest that such comparisons will also offer support for the principal hypotheses tested within it. Another potentially fruitful avenue of investigation would involve cross-sectional and longitudinal comparisons of children who exhibit the NLD syndrome and who are grouped according to the etiology that appears to have produced the syndrome. In this way, differences may emerge between the manifestations of NLD in various types of neurological disease, disorder, and dysfunction.

Two of the limitations of this preliminary investigation are (1) a combination of cross-sectional and longitudinal data were employed in it and (2) only group data for the younger and older subjects were analyzed. Hence, it would be advisable to study single cases over protracted periods of time, in order to determine the viability of the hypotheses in individual cases studied within a longitudinal context. One previously published case (Rourke, Bakker, et al., 1983, pp. 247–253) outlines in some detail the types of preservation and deterioration of skills and abilities that are expected in such persons, and that were also demonstrated in this exploratory investigation. Additional examples of such cases are presented in Chapter 7.

MANIFESTATIONS OF NLD IN NEUROPATHOLOGICAL CONDITIONS

Although we isolated the NLD syndrome in studies that were geared to the determination of the neuropsychological and socioemotional capacities and deficits of children chosen solely on the basis of their presenting profile of academic learning skills (group A), it became clear that children whom we had examined for other reasons also exhibited this syndrome. The groups of children with various forms of neurological disease, disorder, and dysfunction who manifest this syndrome most exactly are listed as follows, with citations of our own case studies and the research reports of some others appearing in parentheses:

1. Many children with moderate to severe head injuries who are able to undergo a comprehensive neuropsychological investigation (Ewing-Cobbs, Fletcher, & Levin, 1985; Fletcher & Levin, 1988)
2. Most children with a hydrocephalic condition that was not treated promptly and/or with success (Rourke, Bakker, et al., 1983, pp. 290–297; Rourke, Fisk, & Strang, 1986, pp. 59–68)
3. Survivors of acute lymphocytic leukemia and other forms of childhood cancer who had received very large doses (treatments) of x-irradiation over a prolonged period of time (Copeland et al., 1985; Fletcher & Copeland, 1988; Rourke, Fisk, & Strang, 1986, pp. 108–116; Taylor, Albo, Phebus, Sachs, & Bierl, 1987)
4. Children with congenital absence of the corpus callosum and who exhibit no other demonstrable neurological disease process (see case study in Rourke, 1987, and in this work, Chapter 7)
5. Children with significant tissue removal from the right cerebral hemisphere (Rourke, Bakker, et al., 1983, pp. 230–238)[1]

It should be pointed out that all of these types of cerebral lesions involve significant destruction or disturbance of function of white matter (long myelinated fibers) in the brain, although the mechanisms of destruction and/or disturbance differ significantly (e.g., *shearing* in the case of the head-injured child, *absence* in the case of children with corpus callosum agenesis, and *removal of tissue* within the right hemisphere).

---

[1]Children and adolescents whose clinical pictures bear a striking resemblance to the social and behavioral characteristics of the NLD child include children with Turner's syndrome (Rourke, Fisk, & Strang, 1986, pp. 136–143), Asperger's syndrome (Baron, 1987; Stevens & Moffitt, 1988; Wing, 1981), Williams syndrome (MacDonald & Roy, 1988), Fragile-X syndrome (Cicchetti, Sparrow, & Rourke, in press), and the so-called "inadequate–immature" delinquent described by Quay (1972). Similar manifestations are also apparent in many persons who exhibit brain impairment as a result of AIDS and the leukodystrophies. Many children afflicted with cerebral palsy (CP) of perinatal, as opposed to postperinatal, etiology would also be expected to manifest the NLD syndrome. However, the large number of neurological abnormalities lumped under the rubric of CP necessitate the separate treatment of this group of disorders. Some considerations of children and adolescents who present with these types of disorders will be dealt with following a discussion of the NLD model.

With respect to lesions affecting large portions of the right cerebral hemisphere, it should be emphasized that much destruction of white matter is quite probable in such instances. This is so because the ratio of white matter to grey matter is much larger in the right cerebral hemisphere than in the left cerebral hemisphere (Goldberg & Costa, 1981; see also Chapter 4 herein)—that is, there is considerably less grey matter relative to white matter in the right than in the left cerebral hemisphere.

Having detailed the characteristics, dynamics, and developmental manifestations of the NLD syndrome, we turn in the next chapter to defining a model by which these processes can be explained.

CHAPTER SIX

The Rourke NLD Right←→Left, Down←→Up, Back←→Front Model (1987/1988)

In order to expand the generalizability and explanatory potential of the Rourke Right→Left Model (1982), it was felt necessary to formulate an extension of this model that would focus on differences and interactions between white and grey matter in the brain. In so doing, an attempt was made to incorporate the down←→up and back←→front neurodevelopmental dimensions that were not considered in the Rourke (1982) model. The resulting expansion of the model, which I have titled the Rourke Right←→Left, Down←→Up, Back←→Front Model (Rourke, 1987, 1988b), would appear to be particularly helpful in the explication of the development of abilities and deficits in at least one well-defined subtype of learning disability, group A. At the same time, this extension was designed to encompass a relatively broad range of the neuropsychological dimensions of human development and their ramifications in aspects of personal, academic, and social functioning. A brief review of some of the salient features of the Goldberg and Costa (1981) and Rourke (1982) models would be helpful as an introduction to this new model.

BACKGROUND

The Goldberg and Costa (1981) model is based primarily upon data gathered and speculations derived from investigations of human adults. Its principal developmental dimension is its emphasis upon the progressive left-hemisphere lateralization of functions throughout the life-span. The Rourke (1982) model was an attempt to expand the elements of this model to encompass early developmental phenomena, especially as these relate to the etiology, course, and persistence of central processing deficiencies in children.

In the Rourke (1982) model, special emphasis was afforded to formulations regarding children who exhibit outstandingly deficient mechanical arithmetic performance relative to word-recognition and spelling performance. Of particular importance in the present context is the fact that these group A children show virtually all of the characteristics of the NLD child. In the Rourke (1982) model it was emphasized that group A children exhibit deficiencies in intermodal integration, problem solving, and concept formation (especially in novel situations), and that they have profound difficulty in benefiting from experiences that do not mesh well with their only existing well-developed, overlearned descriptive system (i.e., natural language). In terms of the formulations of the Goldberg and Costa (1981) model, it was hypothesized that these children exhibit deficient right-hemisphere capacities within a context of well-developed, modality-specific, intramodal, routinized, and stereotyped left-hemisphere skills.

It was emphasized that the deficiencies shown by these children in tactile-perceptual, visual-spatial, visual-perceptual, and psychomotor capacities (deficits that are assumed to have been present from their earliest years) within a context of adequate auditory-perceptual and (eventually) verbal expressive capacities, would be expected to alter substantially the normal course of their development of sensorimotor skills. In turn, it was thought probable that this state of affairs would contribute to considerable developmental deviation in their acquisition of cognitive skills. Specifically, it was thought that their problems in establishing cause-and-effect relationships on a physical, concrete basis during infancy and early childhood would be expected to limit their capacity to develop more abstract levels of thought. Furthermore, this constellation of deficiencies was viewed as causative vis-à-vis the academic and social learning disabilities that these children eventually develop. (The dynamics of the NLD syndrome outlined in Chapter 5 constitute, essentially, a systematic expansion of the interplay of these features first proposed in the 1982 model.)

As an explanation for this state of affairs, it was hypothesized that such children could have deficient right-hemisphere systems and/or insufficient access to initially intact right-hemisphere systems. This level of model development was felt to be sufficient to account for the differences that were evident in the neurodevelopmental course and neuropsychological profiles of the group A youngster (i.e., one manifestation of the NLD syndrome), as compared to those who exhibited other patterns of central processing abilities and deficits.

What is attempted in this chapter is an extension of the Goldberg and Costa (1981) and Rourke (1982) models to account for the specific aspects of early and subsequent neuropsychological development within those domains that are thought to characterize *all* children who exhibit the NLD syndrome.

MAIN THEORETICAL PRINCIPLES AND DEDUCTIONS

The primary theoretical principles upon which an explanation of the phenomena of NLD in children appear to rest are as follows, couched in terms of three principal dimensions of the NLD model: amount of destruction/dysfunction; developmental stage of destruction/dysfunction; development and maintenance of learned behavior.

Amount of White Matter Destroyed or Dysfunctional. In general, the more white matter (relative to total brain mass) that is lesioned, removed, or dysfunctional, the more likely it is that the NLD syndrome will be in evidence. (This is reminiscent of the "mass action" hypothesis of Lashley, 1938.)

Type and Developmental Stage of Destruction or Dysfunction. Which white matter is lesioned, removed, or dysfunctional and at which stage of development this occurs have an important bearing on the manifestations of the NLD syndrome. [This formulation is in clear contradistinction to Lashley's (1938) notion of strict equipotentiality.]

Development and Maintenance of Learned Behavior. Right-hemisphere white matter is crucial for the *development* and *maintenance* of its specific functions, such as intermodal integration, especially when novel information processing situations are encountered. For example, significant destruction or permanent disruption of right-hemisphere white matter would be expected to pose a permanent handicap to the acquisition of new descriptive systems at any developmental stage.

Left-hemisphere white matter is essential for the *development* but not necessarily the *maintenance* of its specific penchants. For example, isolable linguistic skills are often found to remain intact after significant damage to the left cerebral hemisphere in adults. In terms of the model under consideration, once natural language is acquired and automatized, specific functions presumably subserved by the prominent opercula of the left hemisphere would be expected to be relatively impervious to destruction or permanent disruption of white matter not immediately adjacent to and/or forming an integral part of the functioning of these opercula. However, it would be expected that significant disruption of white matter within the left hemisphere during early ontogenetic stages would hamper or even prevent the development of language in the child.

These theoretical principles lead to the following deductions:

Sufficiency. A significant lesion confined to the right cerebral hemisphere may constitute a *sufficient* condition for the production of the NLD syndrome.

Necessity. The *necessary* (and "dose-sensitive") condition for the production of the NLD syndrome is the destruction or dysfunction of white matter that is required for intermodal integration. For example, a significant reduction of callosal fibers or any other neuropathological state that interferes substantially with "access" to right-hemisphere systems—and thus to those systems that are necessary for intermodal integration—would be expected to eventuate in the NLD syndrome.

WHITE MATTER

At this point it would be well to describe briefly the three principal types of white matter fibers that there are in the brain. In the following, a designation regarding the three principal axes of neurodevelopment is employed for each type of white matter:

1. Commissural Fibers (Right ⟷ Left). These nerve fibers cross the midline and interconnect similar regions in the two cerebral hemispheres. There are three sets of such fibers: the corpus callosum, made up of fibers that radiate to interconnect the left and right homologous regions of the frontal, parietal, temporal, and occipital lobes; the anterior, posterior, and habenular commissures; and the hippocampal commissural fibers, of which there are very few in humans. By far the largest set of these fibers is that which constitutes the corpus callosum.

2. *Association Fibers* (*Back* ⟷ *Front*). These are fibers that interconnect cortical regions of the same cerebral hemisphere. They are classified as short association or arcuate fibers, connecting adjacent convolutions within the hemisphere, and long association fibers, connecting cortical regions of the different lobes within the same hemisphere.

3. *Projection Fibers* (*Up* ⟷ *Down*). These fibers project from the diencephalon to the cerebral hemispheres and from the hemispheres to the diencephalon, the brain stem, and the spinal cord. The internal capsule, which handles the "input-output" of the hemispheres, contains projection fibers.

All of these fibers, of course, can be destroyed or rendered dysfunctional by various sorts of neurological disease; however, there are some observations that should be made at this point regarding the *probability* of destruction or disorder within these various types of white matter. First, it is clear that general white matter disease would be expected, by definition, to affect all three types of white matter, with consequent negative impact on all three of the principal axes of neural development.

Second, conditions such as hydrocephalus would be expected to have their principal effects upon commissural (right ⟶ left) and projection (down ⟷ up) fibers, leaving associational (back ⟷ front) fibers relatively intact.

Third, a disease that affects the callosal fibers would be expected to interfere with right-hemisphere ⟷ left-hemisphere "communication." Such a disease would be expected to have a more profound effect upon the functioning of the right hemisphere than the left, because of the right-hemisphere's greater "dependence" upon white matter functioning, especially with regard to its apparent "specialization" for the intermodal integration of novel stimuli. On the other hand, left-hemisphere systems, many of which are relatively "encapsulated" within the three major opercula (grey matter and short association fibers) may maintain enough stimulation within and between each other so that some fairly sophisticated intramodal integrations can proceed with little or no input from the right cerebral hemisphere. The upshot of all of this is that left-hemisphere systems are probably able to function reasonably well in the face of callosal and projection fiber damage, so long as association fibers are intact. Even in the latter instance, however, intact associational fibers would appear to be necessary for the *development* but not for the *maintenance* of left-hemisphere functioning.

One deduction that can be made from this state of affairs is that one would expect to see the principal (primary, secondary, and tertiary) neuropsychological features of the NLD syndrome *plus* global linguistic deficiencies (as in autism) only if there is early associational fiber disease within the left cerebral hemisphere *plus* white matter disease that affects intermodal integration. Associational fiber destruction, disorder, or dysfunction in the left hemisphere *after* natural language has been acquired should lead to aphasia (of the conduction or similar varieties) but not to autism. (These ideas will be expanded upon later.)

It is my expectation that close clinical neuropsychological monitoring of children and adolescents with the various types of neurological disease, disorder, and dysfunction referred to here will eventuate in profiles characterized as being typical of the NLD child. Investigation of children and adolescents with neuropsychiatric disorders, the published accounts of which bear a striking resemblance to the manifestations of the NLD syndrome (e.g., those who exhibit Asperger's syndrome, alexithymia, and/or inadequate/immature types of delinquency), would be expected to yield similar findings. In addition, it is my expectation that, in the future, studies employing sophisticated neural imaging techniques that are capable of assessing metabolic changes during central processing tasks will eventually demonstrate that the white matter versus grey matter relationships suggested in this model are causative with respect to the NLD syndrome.

GENERAL DEVELOPMENTAL IMPLICATIONS

Integrity of white matter (long myelinated fiber) function would appear to be necessary for the *development* of systems within both hemispheres and crucial for both the *development* and the *maintenance* of those functions subserved primarily by systems within the right hemispheral systems, but not necessary for the *maintenance* of some functions subserved primarily by systems within the left hemisphere.

The NLD syndrome would be expected to develop under any set of circumstances that interferes significantly with the functioning of right-hemisphere systems, as in the case of any general deterioration of white matter or with substantial destruction of white matter within the right hemisphere, and/or access to neuronal intercommunication with these systems, as in the case of callosal agenesis.

Furthermore, the likelihood that the NLD syndrome will be manifest is increased by any neurological disease that has the effect of "isolating"—from each other and/or from right-hemisphere systems—one or more of the three prominent opercula of the left hemisphere that play a crucial role in its essentially intramodal functions of routinization and stereotypic application of previously acquired descriptive systems (e.g., natural language). Such a scenario would effectively handicap the affected individuals in the acquisition of new descriptive systems and would increase the likelihood that they would apply previously acquired descriptive systems in a rigid, stereotyped, perseverative fashion within situations where such application is not necessarily adaptive. The set of phenomena associated with normal aging may be one example of such a state of affairs; symptoms associated with advanced stages of any number of demylenating diseases may be another. It should be noted that, for both of these examples, a *general* deterioration in white matter, rather than a *specific* deterioration of left-hemisphere white matter, would be expected to be the rule rather than the exception.

In any case, the loss of the capacity to generate new descriptive systems helps to explain the essentially downward course over successive developmental epochs that is observed in individuals who manifest the NLD syndrome. Considering the entire developmental course of this syndrome, it would seem that it is less apparent at the age of 7 to 8 years (Ozols & Rourke, 1988, in press) than at 10 to 14 years (Rourke & Finlayson, 1978; Rourke & Strang, 1978; Strang & Rourke, 1983), and that it becomes progressively more apparent (and more debilitating) as adulthood approaches (Rourke, Bakker, et al., 1983, pp. 247–253; Rourke, Young, et al., 1986).

In connection with this last observation, it should be noted that formal operational thought (a feature of higher-order cognitive functioning that is notably deficient in older children and adolescents who manifest the NLD syndrome) is not within the developmental capacities of the 7- to 8-year-old child. Since it becomes a developmental task/demand as the child approaches puberty—and, of course, increases in adaptive importance as the individual progresses through adolescence and into adulthood—it should come as no surprise that progressive deterioration in skills associated with such capacities (e.g., socioemotional adaptation) is the rule rather than the exception. Evidence of such deterioration is apparent in the cross-sectional and longitudinal studies of such individuals cited earlier in this book.

THEORETICAL AND CLINICAL IMPLICATIONS

The heuristic implications of this explanatory model may be seen best in specific instances of the presence or absence of the NLD syndrome in various forms of neurological disease, disorder, and dysfunction. In the examples that follow, an attempt is made to address the theoretical and clinical dimensions, generalizations, explanations, and predictions that would be consistent with the elements of the model. Comments on the role of the model in assessment of various neurological disease processes and suggestions regarding empirical tests of the model are highlighted.

General or Diffuse Destruction of White Matter

The neurological diseases and disorders just mentioned that eventuate in the NLD syndrome do so to the extent that they involve destruction of white matter; the more white matter that is destroyed or permanently disordered, the more likely it is that the syndrome will be manifest. This would be expected to be especially the case in conditions that involve general or diffuse destruction of white matter, such as may result from intensive or extensive radiotherapy of the brain or extensive white matter shearing, as in significant craniocerebral trauma following acceleration-deceleration injuries. In this connection, Taylor, Albo, Phebus, Sachs, and Bieri (1987) showed that, in elementary school children who survived acute lymphocytic leukemia (ALL), higher doses of brain radiation used to prevent or treat the disease were associated with lower IQ scores (WISC-R Full Scale and Performance IQs), poorer neuropsychological performances (tests of eye–hand coordination and visual-motor integration), and greater difficulties in school as judged by parent ratings and by special help received. Furthermore, the ALL group as a whole in this study exhibited a pattern of relatively high scores on the WRAT Reading and Spelling subtests, as compared to their performance on the WRAT Arithmetic subtest. Similar conclusions have been arrived at by Fletcher and Copeland (1988) in their review of the ALL literature.

Craniocerebral Trauma

The notion that right-hemisphere skills are more affected than are left-hemisphere skills by significant head injury in children and adults may be a reflection of the state of affairs outlined just above. Consistent with this view are the observations of Taylor (1984, 1987), who cites a variety of sources of evidence to suggest that children who sustain brain injury early in life exhibit their greatest impairments on tests of visual-motor skill, problem solving, memory and learning, and psychomotor and mental efficiency. He also points out that tasks requiring uncomplicated and possibly overpracticed verbal responses appear to be the least compromised by such injury.

In addition, it would be consistent with our clinical observations and with the elements of the model under consideration that those children who are likely to have been most at risk for sustaining head injuries (e.g., as a result of not anticipating the consequences of their actions) are those who, prior to their injury, exhibit the NLD syndrome. Hence, it should come as no surprise that they appear to be so subsequent to their injury, which can explain the often-noted finding of lower WISC Performance IQ relative to Verbal IQ following significant craniocerebral trauma (Rutter, 1982). In the case of children who, after a normal course of development, suffer some *general* deterioration in white matter with consequent manifestations of the NLD syndrome, a similar state of affairs would be expected to obtain, that is, a manifestation of relative deterioration of abilities and skills ordinarily thought to be subserved primarily by right-hemisphere systems and relative sparing of those thought to be mediated by left-hemisphere systems.

As just mentioned, it is common to find the characteristics of the NLD syndrome evident in persons who have suffered significant craniocerebral trauma and who have recovered to the point where they are able to undergo a comprehensive neuropsychological assessment. In addition to the NLD characteristics, such persons may exhibit two other sets of significant deficits, namely, those that appear to be related to general attentional deployment and focal (cortical grey matter) contusion. With these variables in mind, the following formulation of the deficits following significant craniocerebral trauma—hereafter referred to as closed head injury, or CHI—would seem appropriate: $CHI = AD + NLD + FD$. In this equation, AD stands for attentional deficit (i.e., arousal system disturbance), NLD stands for nonverbal learning disabilities syndrome (i.e., reflections of white matter disease), and FD stands for focal disturbance (i.e., grey matter contusion).

Two "ingredients" of this formulation are commonly acknowledged sequelae of severe head injury. For example, it has been known for some time that attentional deficit is a frequent result of CHI. It is also common knowledge that persons undergoing significant CHI, especially in acceleration–deceleration situations, may suffer from focal disturbances occasioned by grey matter lesions, especially in the anterior temporal and frontal regions of the brain. What is new about this formulation is the specification of the characteristics of the NLD syndrome. There would appear to be some advantages of the latter for the assessment of CHI patients, as the following is meant to suggest.

Let us start with attentional deficit or arousal disturbances. In the main, these are *general* disturbances of attentional deployment that affect virtually all types of performance. (These should be distinguished from the *modality-specific* attentional deficits that form part of the NLD syndrome.) The slowing of response occasioned by such general attentional disturbances is most often seen in situations that involve complex choice reaction time and in other decision-making situations (Van Zomeren, 1981). If attentional deficit of significant proportions does not clear with the passage of time, there is little likelihood that the NLD syndrome and/or the effects of any focal disturbance of grey matter will be reflected in neuropsychological test results with any degree of clarity.[1]

However, if the general attentional deficit subsides sufficiently for a comprehensive neuropsychological examination to be conducted and, indeed, if it subsides to the point where it poses little or no adaptive problems for the patient, we are in a position to examine the other two "ingredients" of CHI: the NLD syndrome and focal disturbance. Figure 6.1 illustrates how the latter can be deduced, using the equation just described.

Consider first the graphs for the NLD syndrome, the data for which, at present, are theoretical. They do, however, represent the average performance of the approximately 11-year-old children in group A who were included in the studies reviewed in Chapter 2. Also included in this

[1]This situation prompted the analogy of "psychic edema" (Rourke, 1983b), which is inferred to characterize the performance of young brain-damaged children; when this psychic edema, which manifests behaviorally as an attentional deficit, clears with the passing of time, one is able to see the effects of focal disturbance (e.g., linguistic disturbances of particular types) that, although present all along, do not show up until the "edema" subsides.

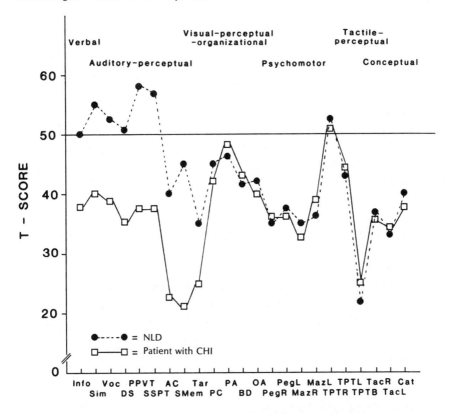

FIGURE 6.1. Mean *T* scores for 11-year-old NLD children compared with those for an 11-year-old child with CHI. A *T* score of 50 reflects the mean performance for normal 11-year-olds on the tests within each of the six categories. Performances on each of the 23 variables within these categories are arranged such that good performance is represented by *T* scores above 50 and poor performance is represented by *T* scores less than 50. For explanation of abbreviations, see legend to Figure 2.1.

figure is a set of hypothetical neuropsychological test results for an 11-year-old child who has suffered a severe CHI. It is assumed that this child was able to undergo this examination, which means that there would have been at least partial clearing of the general attentional deficit that followed the injury. The inference that I would suggest can be made in this instance is that the *difference* between the patient's neuropsychological profile and the NLD profile appropriate for his age is the result of focal disturbance. In other words, being able to hypothesize the typical

NLD test results, while assuming minimal attentional deficit, allows one to attribute the remaining differences to focal disturbance.

An obvious requirement for the utilization of this method for inferring focal disturbance is to have age-appropriate NLD profiles with which to compare individual test results. Because of the decline in some areas (e.g., concept formation and problem solving) inferred with advancing years, it is clear that such developmental profiles are needed.

My reasons for suggesting that the adoption of this procedure may be helpful in the clinical situation relate not only to the generating of inferences per se (which might be confirmed through neuro-imaging or other techniques), but also to the fact that neuroradiologists often prefer to have some indication of the site of the focal disturbance in question. Such an inference may justify taking a closer look (i.e., taking more "cuts") of a particular brain region than would ordinarily be the case. Enhanced specification of the lesion may then be possible. More generally, however, it is often helpful to know that there are particular behavioral deficits that are present that are quite different from the NLD presentation; these may (and probably do) require quite different forms of intervention than those that are found helpful in dealing with the manifestations of NLD.

Neurotoxins and the Cortical versus Subcortical Dementias

The notion that many toxic substances and teratogens have different effects upon the "developing" organism than upon the "mature" organism may also be a reflection of the mechanisms envisioned in connection with general or diffuse destruction of white matter and craniocerebral trauma. That is, those substances in large quantities that are known to affect white matter more than grey matter would be expected to have a *general* effect on all aspects of behavior in the immature organism, but relatively more *specific* effects in the adult, such as on abilities and skills more dependent upon intact right-hemisphere systems. In fact, it may be heuristic to reverse this cause-and-effect relationship; that is, it may be fruitful to investigate hypotheses regarding differential effects upon white and grey matter of certain toxic substances as a function of the skills and abilities that are seen to be impaired by them at different stages of development.

This is not the place to review the literature dealing with the distinction between cortical and subcortical dementias or that dealing with the effects of various environmental toxins on brain substance and behavior. What is relevant here is a consideration of the manner in which the tenets of the NLD model might be put to empirical test. The relevant experimental design in this instance is quite simple, as the following examples should illustrate.

First, older adults who are carrying a diagnosis of dementia could be differentiated into those who are suffering from a cortical as opposed to a subcortical dementia. Once technical difficulties in neuro-imaging techniques (such as the "partial-volume" problem) are resolved, this differentiation could then be verified with the aid of positron emission tomography (PET), cerebral blood flow, and other methods. All subjects would undergo a comprehensive neuropsychological investigation that would include measures of skills and abilities that are hypothesized to be assets and deficits in the NLD syndrome. The experimental hypotheses under investigation would be quite straightforward:

1. Persons exhibiting verified subcortical dementia should exhibit a pattern of assets and deficits that is similar to the NLD syndrome.
2. The extent to which the NLD syndrome is manifest in such patients should be a fairly direct reflection of the *amount* of white matter that has been destroyed or rendered dysfunctional.
3. Specific subtypes of subcortical dementia would be expected as a function of the site(s) of white matter destruction or dysfunction.
4. Persons with dementia that is verified to be exclusively of cortical origin would not be expected to exhibit the NLD syndrome.

Were younger persons to be involved in this experimental design, one would anticipate some effects as a result of the time of onset of the dementia; however, this will not concern us here.

In addition, some neurotoxins are known to affect white matter more than grey matter. This being the case, one could carry out systematic comparisons of individuals who have been exposed to such toxins and who have had the brain lesions resulting from such exposure verified by the types of brain-imaging techniques just mentioned. A comprehensive neuropsychological assessment of such individuals should reflect findings, *mutatis mutandis*, in accord with all four of the preceding hypotheses.

More generally, it would be expected that the NLD syndrome would manifest in persons who were suffering from white matter disease or dysfunction, and that the extent of the manifestations of the syndrome would be a fairly direct reflection of the amount of white matter that had been destroyed or was disordered or dysfunctional. More subtle nuances to this scenario would involve acute versus insidious onset of white matter disease and the developmental stage at which it was suffered. The latter will be addressed in conjunction with the case presentations in Chapter 7.

Aphasia

White matter destruction in some areas of the left cerebral hemisphere (e.g., as seen in the "disconnection syndrome") does not eventuate in global aphasia in the adult who has previously acquired and automatized natural language. Prior to such acquisition and automatization (e.g., in early infancy), however, substantial destruction or permanent disruption of white matter within the left cerebral hemisphere may prevent the acquisition of language. In neither of these cases would one expect to see the manifestations of the NLD syndrome. This syndrome is expected to occur only if the child's or the adult's intermodal integration capacities are interfered with. Hence, in cases where there is significant disruption of left-hemisphere white matter but sparing of the corpus callosum, projection fiber, and right-hemisphere associational white matter, various forms of aphasia or developmental language disorder would be expected to occur, in the absence of manifestations of the NLD syndrome.

Autism

There are several important facts about autism that have a bearing on the application of the NLD model in an attempt to deal with the etiology and manifestations of autism. Two of these are as follows:

1. Adults do not become autistic following brain lesions or under any other stressful circumstance.
2. Adults can manifest the NLD syndrome, however, as a result of a number of neurological disease processes, including brain lesions involving significant portions of the right cerebral hemisphere, closed head injury, and extensive white matter disease resulting from any number of factors. Normal aging and perhaps some of the so-called subcortical dementias also appear to have this syndrome as one of their correlates.

As an explanation for these two facts, it should be noted that, in the NLD model, it is inferred that white matter is necessary for the development of skills mediated by many left-hemisphere systems, but that it is not necessary for their maintenance. Thus, if white matter is present and functional during the early development of language and other skills that come to be mediated—and therefore automatized—by left-hemisphere systems, subsequent lesions of white matter can be quite profound while these skills would still be expected to remain relatively functional. The most obvious cases in point are the "crystallized" skills of language— skills that, once established, are all but impervious to many perturbations of white matter function. Notice in all of this that such skills are not impervious to significant lesions of the three principal opercula (clumps of grey matter) within the left cerebral hemisphere, which can be expected to have devastating effects on various aspects of language. Indeed, one would expect that the more automatized (i.e., the better developed) the linguistic skills, the more devastating the consequences that would be expected to ensue with such lesions. In addition, in the case of significant lesions of associational fibers within the left hemisphere of the mature brain, it is possible to observe many intact linguistic functions within the general picture of the "disconnection" syndrome and related aphasiologic presentations (see Chapter 2 of Rourke, Fisk, & Strang, 1986).

This is one example of a more general principle of brain–behavior relationships: The more specialized any particular area is for the mediation of a particular set of skills or abilities, the more devastating the consequences for such skills or abilities when this area is destroyed. The architecture of the left cerebral hemisphere is best seen as composed of, on the one hand, such highly specialized areas (clumps of grey matter) and, on the other hand, areas that, over the course of development, become progressively less necessary for the satisfactory functioning of these specialized areas. The right hemisphere, by contrast, is seen as more diffuse and interrelated in its functioning. Although this is not meant to suggest that the right hemisphere is composed of "equipotential" systems, it is suggested that its neurological architecture is such that lesions in a wide variety of areas can very often result in similar, if not almost identical, behavioral sequelae (see Kertesz & Dobrowolski, 1981).

Returning to the example of autism, there are at least two questions that have a bearing on this matter: If early white matter damage is thought to be so devastating to the early acquisition of all skills, why would a condition such as congenital callosal agenesis not eventuate in autism? By the same token, why would early hydrocephalus, which is known to cause damage to periventricular white matter, not eventuate in autism?

In answer to these questions, it should be noted that much of the damage to white matter in callosal agenesis and hydrocephalus is completely or largely confined to the white matter that serves to *connect* the two cerebral hemispheres, and in some cases to projection fibers. Much, if not the great majority, of *intra*hemispheric (associational fiber) white matter is preserved in both of these conditions. This would suggest that very little *inter*hemispheric white matter is necessary in order to develop many aspects of language. Children with callosal agenesis and various types and degrees of hydrocephalus often develop the NLD syndrome. They quite characteristically develop the first aspects of language late in development but quickly attain the more rote, prosaic aspects of language at age-appropriate or better levels and rates. It may be the case in autism that *intra*hemispheric (associational) white matter tracts are destroyed or rendered dysfunctional during a very early developmental period, possibly well before birth. This might occur in conjunction with *inter*hemispheric white matter tract damage. Damage to callosal fibers would not be either necessary or sufficient, however, to eventuate in the complete absence of linguistic development. It would be sufficient to lead to the type of linguistic development that characterizes the NLD syndrome, namely, good rote language skills and impoverished pragmatics and content.

It is hypothesized that autistic children who eventually develop language will be shown to have some intrahemispheric (associational) white matter tracts within the left cerebral hemisphere that are intact. This would account for the development of some language. Their autistic features would be expected to result from extensive damage to interhemispheric (callosal) and/or right-hemisphere intrahemispheric (associational) and/or projection fiber white matter tracts. In these scenarios, right-hemisphere systems would be either dysfunctional, or unreachable, or grossly understimulated (and thus, eventually, dysfunctional).

There are three other features of autism that may be clarified with reference to the NLD model: echolalia; pronominal reversal; and an apparent fear of novelty, with consequent attraction to sameness. Echolalia would imply some connectivity within the left hemisphere. Perhaps the problem in language development for those who exhibit echolalia is difficulty in tying words to meanings. In turn, this may be caused by a lack of access to right-hemisphere systems. The frequent presence of pronominal reversal (e.g., the use of *me* for *you*) may also be an example of the latter. It should be noted that this effect is *constant*; that is, the autistic child always uses the same formula for this reversal. This would imply an overautomatization of response, a feature of the NLD syndrome that is inferred to result from white matter disease, disorder, or dysfunction that interferes with intermodal integration.

Finally, the desire for sameness may be another example of overautomatization. What appears to be a fear of novelty in the autistic child may reflect an inability to countenance novelty, a basic neuropsychological deficit that is inferred to play a significant role in the NLD syndrome. Perhaps the inability to put into words the stimulus changes that are apparent (e.g., a chair where the television "should" be) also plays a role here. But, what is the neuropsychological basis for aversion for novelty? An answer to this question that is within the context of the NLD model and has some general applicability is as follows.

It is expected that the autistic child will develop some elementary although grossly inflexible codes. It would seem probable, however, that the codes that the mute autistic child does manage to develop will not have the opportunity to become automatized. This is so because the white matter (associational fiber) connections in the left hemisphere are deficient. One result of this lack of automatization is that the child would constantly have to deal with old situations (i.e., ones that should be familiar) as though they were new. This would be expected to generate a considerable amount of stress and anxiety in the child, which may be avoided by adopting a perceptual set that reduces novelty. This could be accomplished by employing a single visual–spatial template of the "old" and effectively altering new stimulus situations to make them fit the old. In this way, the child essentially assimilates every new situation in terms of a single old one. This lack of suitable accommodation to the new is inferred to result from an inability to automatize codes. Were the latter possible for the autistic child, the end result would be a reduction in the anxiety that is generated by constantly having to address every environmental presentation as a novel event.

This situation is analogous to the normal infant's emerging "fear" of strangers. Although having developed the capacity to differentiate the old (familiar) from the new (novel), the infant is not yet capable of automatizing (i.e., categorizing or filing) the new in terms of preexisting categories, such as friend, foe, mean person, and so on. Once the infant is able to do this routinely, fear of strangers should disappear. This is not at all meant to imply that the child's categorization of such persons is correct; rather, the child infers that the categorization is correct and, if the categorization is benign, does not feel fear. It is clear that parents must often teach their children to be fearful of strangers. This is so because the child may very well infer that all persons are nice or good. In this sense, the parent is encouraging the development of flexible categorization as the best means for insuring adequate adaptation to situations that pose a potential threat to the child. The important point with respect to the NLD model in this instance is the fact that more flexible categorizations rest upon the automatization of more elementary perceptions, and that each level of this type of cognitive advance must be automatized, at least to a certain extent, before more advanced levels can be obtained. (For an example of this phenomenon in the learning-to-read process, see Chapter 4.) The important feature of the autistic child's cognitive development here is the failure to transcend very primitive levels of automatization, possibly as a result of a combination of deficits in intermodal (right-hemisphere) and intramodel (left-hemisphere) integration.

By way of summary, a possible mechanism for early infantile autism may be the absence of sufficient white matter to connect the principal opercula of the left cerebral hemisphere in the early phases of language acquisition. Indeed, the positive correlation between the amount of language in autistic children and their eventual social/adaptive outcome may reflect various points on a gradient of white matter disease or dysfunction in this disorder (or continuum of disorders). For example, it may be the case that mute autistic children are bereft of even those minimal associational fibers that are necessary for some linguistic development to take place. But, even in those with some language attainment, there are indications of extreme difficulties in social relationships, including poor social judgment and socially inappropriate behavior. This state of affairs would suggest that it is quite likely that there is a *general* condition of white matter deterioration in the autistic syndrome, rather than one that is confined to the left hemisphere. It is also the case that the autistic syndrome would be expected to be manifest when there is widespread dysfunction of the white matter in the right hemisphere from the very earliest ontogenetic stages. This would be expected to hamper the attainment of all descriptive systems, including natural language, as well as to produce the principal deficiencies that characterize the NLD syndrome. It would appear, however, that such dysfunction would have to be quite severe and/or widespread if natural language were to be completely absent.

At the same time, this explanatory model would suggest that a similar extreme deficiency in white matter functioning in the adult would *not* be expected to eventuate in anything approaching the manifestations of the autistic syndrome. Clearly, this is the case in adults suffering from significant white matter disease: Adults do not develop anything approaching full-blown autistic manifestations. In terms of the model under consideration, this would be expected to be the case because previously normal adults would have already acquired a number of descriptive systems that could be applied in an easy fashion to a large number of vocational and interpersonal situations, as a result of their automatization of linguistic skills through the agency of grey matter intensive structures within the left cerebral hemisphere. In fact, the behavioral and other manifestations of diffuse white matter disease with adult onset may provide the basis for a working model regarding neuropsychological differences between early and late dysfunction of white matter.

It should be clear that the proposed inclusion of autism under the umbrella of the NLD syndrome is quite contrary to the suggestions of Fein, Pennington, Markowitz, Braverman, and Waterhouse (1986), and others, to the effect that social deficits may be *primary* in the set of disabilities included under the rubric of autism. Viewed from the perspective of the NLD syndrome and model, social and other adaptional deficits are, quite unequivocally, the *effect* rather than the *cause* of the four types of neuropsychological deficiencies that are posited to lie at their basis. This, of course, ultimately applies to white matter deficiencies as well.

Aging

In senescence, the notion that the right hemisphere ages faster than does the left may be one reflection of an *equal* amount of deterioration of all neurons within both hemispheres with advancing years. This would be the case if, in aging, white matter is more prone to deterioration than is grey matter. If such be the case, it would be predicted that, as the senium approaches, there would be more marked functional/behavioral deficiencies of the particular proclivities of the right hemisphere systems (e.g., dealing with novelty) and relatively more sparing of the penchants of left-hemisphere systems (e.g., automatized language). This would be so because of the higher ratio of white to grey matter in the right hemisphere than in the left, and the necessity for more connectivity in the right hemisphere in order to meet the requirements for intermodal integration.

Any general deterioration of white matter is likely to yield evidence of more deterioration in fluid than in crystallized abilities. To the extent that the aging process or any other condition that is likely to eventuate in such general deterioration of white matter (e.g., prolonged alcoholism) obtains the more probable it becomes that symptoms thought to be indicative of right-hemisphere dysfunction will appear. In fact, this would probably be best characterized as a "functional" lateralized disturbance which reflects *more* disturbance of right-hemisphere functioning and probably mirrors *equal* deterioration of white matter in both cerebral hemispheres.

GENERAL TREATMENT IMPLICATIONS

The preceding discussion of theoretical and clinical implications would suggest strongly that the following principles of treatment for children and adolescents who manifest the NLD syndrome are viable. (These would appear to apply, *mutatis mutandis*, to adults as well.)

First, the earlier in development that white matter disease of significant dimensions occurs, the more propitious it would be to "attack" the deficits of the child in a direct fashion. The rationale for such a principle is fairly straightforward: It would seem reasonable to attempt to stimulate the functioning of the remaining white matter to the maximum, in an effort to encourage the development of centers of grey matter that are dependent upon input from white matter for their adequate development. It is at this time that intensive physiotherapy and related interventions aimed at increasing sensorimotor integration would be expected to be most efficacious. Failure to follow such a program during these early years may lead to "secondary degeneration" of such grey matter (Rourke, Bakker, et al., 1983, p. 178). Perhaps most important, this activity may stimulate those principal clumps of ganglia (opercula) of the left cerebral hemisphere that are crucial for the development of natural language. In any case, during these early stages of development it would seem to be particularly unpropitious to adopt a laissez-faire attitude toward child-rearing with such youngsters; this would essentially encourage them to languish in a neuropsychologically isolated and largely understimulated personal world.

Second, the longer the NLD syndrome persists and the later it occurs in the development of the individual, the more probable it becomes that accentuation of compensatory techniques (e.g., the use of intact rote verbal memory skills) will prove to be efficacious for adaptational and therapeutic purposes. For example, it would appear to be particularly appropriate to encourage the adoption of compensatory strategies for older children who have acquired natural language to an advanced level prior to the onset of significant white matter disease or dysfunction. For such children, the use of compensatory strategies (largely of the verbal variety) for social and vocational adaptation would appear to be one of the very few feasible and efficacious therapeutic/rehabilitational tacks to pursue. (A more specific therapeutic program for persons exhibiting NLD is described in Chapter 7.)

GENERAL CONCLUSIONS

In a first attempt at the formulation of a developmental neuropsychological model aimed at the explication of central processing abilities and deficiencies in children (Rourke, 1982), I emphasized the salience of the right-hemisphere←→left-hemisphere distinction and interactions. I noted at the time that it would eventually become necessary to incorporate the so-called up←→down and front←→back dimensions into this model if it were to constitute a reasonably complete theoretical formulation of developmental neuropsychological functioning. The NDL model, which is an attempt to account for the behavioral consequences of destruction or permanent incapacity of various types of white versus grey matter at various stages of development, is a step in the direction of this more general developmental neuropsychological theory.

In this context, it would appear that Lashley's (1938) formulations regarding *mass action* (remember that he was dealing with lesions in rat brain, where the proportion of white to grey matter is considerably greater than is the case in the human brain) loom large in the explanation of the neurological diseases and developmental learning disabilities under consideration and in what appears to be their final common pathway, the NLD syndrome. That is, it is proposed in the NLD model that positive, "dose-sensitive" (although not necessarily linear) relationships obtain between amount (mass) of brain substance destroyed, disordered, or rendered dysfunctional and the degree of neuropsychological deficit that ensues therefrom. This relationship is inferred to obtain in the case of white, not grey, matter.

At the same time, Lashley's (1938) notion that neurons have equal potential to mediate behavior stands in marked contrast to the formulations enunciated in the NLD model. Indeed, this model points (1) to the necessity for particular, unique, hemisphere-specific, nonsubstitutable processes to be extant and functioning at particular stages of ontogeny if normal development is to proceed and (2) to the abnormal developmental consequences that are thought to ensue if such be not the case.

QUESTIONS OFTEN ASKED REGARDING
THE NLD SYNDROME AND MODEL

Why Is This Syndrome Characterized
as a "Learning Disability"?

In addition to the obvious fact that the NLD syndrome was isolated within the context of research attempts aimed at the specification of reliable and valid subtypes of learning disabilities, there are four very important reasons for considering it within the context of learning disabilities:

1. New learning of any sort, especially in complex or novel situations, is especially difficult for children who exhibit the characteristics of NLD. New learning experiences must be introduced very gradually to such children; they must be apprised verbally of all the elements of the learning situations; these verbal descriptions and elaborations need to be repeated and expanded upon frequently; and the initial phases of the learning process for such children are very slow and laborious.

2. When faced with novel or complex learning requirements, these children quite typically fall back on the use of some overlearned procedure for dealing with the situation, without regard for the unique aspects of the new learning task. This excessive reliance on previously overlearned responses and techniques becomes less and less appropriate as development proceeds. That is, it becomes less and less likely that NLD individuals, left to their own resorts, will learn new or complex task demands in an adequate manner. Instead, there is an increasing tendency toward stereotyped or even perseverative responding. In a word, their problems in benefiting from particular types of stimulus presentations, informational complexity, and appropriate reinforcement in any number of day-to-day situations are clear and obvious.

3. Adaptability is the raison d'être of brain–behavior development. Deficiencies in adaptability are, essentially, deficiencies in learning. In this sense, the rather devastating set of learning problems experienced by the

person who exhibits NLD are among the very worst that can be imagined from a psychological perspective. The social and vocational incompetence, the withdrawal, and the psychic pain are terminal adaptive manifestations of failures of learning. These are all manifestations of the fact that "talk is very cheap" when compared to the richness of adaptive learning.

4. Attempts at remediation with such individuals are generally effective to the extent that they consistently follow well-established guidelines for cognitive-behavioral therapy. It must be emphasized that such therapy should proceed within the context of a full realization and appreciation of the particular proclivities and penchants of the information processing capacities of such persons. (See Chapter 7 for the specifics of such a program.)

What Is the Clinical Incidence of NLD, Relative to Other Learning Disabilities?

Beginning around 1968, when we first carried out neuropsychological examinations of children whom we eventually came to characterize in terms of the NLD rubric, the incidence of NLD in children referred for neuropsychological assessment because of suspected learning disabilities was quite low. For every 20 or so children who exhibited a learning disability first noted in the academic milieu and of apparent psycholinguistic origin, we would see only 1 school-identified child who exhibited NLD. More recently, this ratio has been halved to approximately 1 in 10, and there are indications that this trend toward a higher incidence of NLD is continuing.

Of course, this "trend" is also influenced by the increased quality of treatment that has been afforded to children with acute lymphocytic leukemia, those who suffer severe closed head injuries, and children with the types of neurological disorders wherein the NLD syndrome is quite frequent. Whereas, 20 years ago, many if not most of such children would have expired soon after the onset of the disorder, many if not most now survive. This increase in survival rate raises the incidence of children who present with the NLD syndrome when subjected to a comprehensive neuropsychological evaluation, a form of assessment that is being increasingly seen as a crucial aspect of treatment planning for such children.

It is always hazardous to speculate on clinical statistics, because so many factors can impinge on them. For example, we may be assessing a higher proportion of children with the developmental manifestation of the NLD syndrome because school officials are becoming more adept at (1) dealing with children whose academic learning problems relate to one or more aspects of psycholinguistic skill development and (2) identifying NLD children as being in need of assistance. Evidence in favor of the latter point is the fact that such children are now being referred at much younger ages than was heretofore the case. However, even this may be a function of our community situation and the availability of services for such children. Other factors that may increase the referral to us of children who exhibit NLD characteristics may relate to an increased emphasis on physical education in our area schools over the past 20 years, a greater sensitivity to socioemotional and other adaptational problems on the part of school personnel, and more attention being paid to anxious or withdrawn children, in addition to their more obvious hyperactive or conduct-disordered agemates.

These somewhat "provincial" factors are mentioned in order to alert clinicians to the need to be sensitive to such dimensions in their own communities. Clinical incidence varies markedly between communities, as a function of the quantity, quality, and "profile level" of the clinical services available; the cost of such services; and a host of other sociopolitical factors that can exert profound impacts on referral patterns. Be that as it may, it is felt that the factors that have been raised in conjunction with this question are important ones to consider, and they suggest the more general questions that need to be posed in relation to this matter.

Are There Sex Differences in the Incidence of NLD?

Also around 1968, the sex ratio of children referred to us who manifested NLD characteristics at assessment was approximately one girl for every five or six boys. Now, some 20 years later, we find that the sex ratio is 1:1. It is clear to me that the gender role expectation revolution that has transpired during this period has resulted in this dramatic change in the gender ratio of clinical incidence; it is also apparent that the occurrence of this revolution has eventuated in a clinical incidence that is equivalent to the "true" incidence. Let me explain these two propositions.

First, it is apparent that young girls, at least in Western society, are now expected to engage in roughly the same tasks (i.e., meet the same developmental demands) as do young boys. Girls are expected to engage in vigorous track-and-field events, contact sports, and other endeavors that used to be the almost exclusive domain of boys, with the exception of a few girls referred to as "tomboys" a quarter of a century ago. In addition, girls are expected to do as well as boys in school subjects involving mathematics and science. The gender role revolution has changed dramatically the expectations that society (as reflected principally in the school) has for performance involving motor and psychomotor skills, visual-spatial-organizational skills, concept-formation, and scientific activities. Thus, it should come as no surprise that girls who present with difficulties in these areas (i.e., difficulties of the NLD sort) would be seen, even during the early school years, as in need of some form of assessment and/or intervention. Whereas 20 or more years ago the shy, withdrawn, psychomotorically incompetent girl who had difficulties with arithmetic/mathematics would be thought of as normally demure and essentially "feminine," such is not the case today. Hence, we have experienced a dramatic increase in the incidence of girls being referred for assessment because such characteristics are now viewed as "symptoms" or "problems," rather than "normal" feminine characteristics.

But, why should a ratio of 1:1 be viewed as the *true* incidence rate? There are two sets of answers for this. First, there is no reason to believe that fetal teratogens such as alcohol and other drugs, x-irradiation, and so on should affect the male fetus more or less than the female fetus; birth defects are not appreciably more common in boys than in girls; and given the more vigorous participation of girls in contact sports and in other activities such as motor vehicle driving, one would expect there to be, eventually, an equivalence in the incidence of significant head injuries for both genders. All of these and many more that could be mentioned are factors that can lead to the manifestations of the NLD syndrome. Second, the origins of the NLD syndrome, at this point, would not appear to be related to genetic factors. Even if this were to some extent the case, there is no reason at this point to infer that such genetic factors would be sex linked. For both of these sets of reasons, the "true" incidence of NLD should not be related to gender, either in terms of current gender role expectations or in terms of gender-linked genetic anomalies.

Why Do Patients Suffering from Craniocerebral Trauma Often Present with Features That Suggest Right-Hemisphere Dysfunction?

There are several reasons for this finding, not all of which are mutually exclusive. Some of these are as follows:

1. There is a greater proportion of white to grey matter in the right cerebral hemisphere than in the left. Hence, an event such as significant craniocerebral trauma, which is known to cause extensive white matter shearing, is likely to cause much more damage to the structures and systems of the right hemisphere than of the left.

2. The systems of the right hemisphere are inferred to be principally responsible for intermodal integration and dealing with novel information. Most tests that are thought to be "sensitive" to right-hemisphere functioning (e.g., WISC Block Design) are more novel in nature than are those thought typically to reflect left-hemisphere functioning (e.g., WISC Vocabulary). The latter type of test tends to tap into overlearned, rote, verbal information that is crystallized to the point that it becomes somewhat impervious to general white matter dysfunction. The systems within the right hemisphere are not thought to be specialized for or capable of this sort of intramodal functioning. Thus, if there is general white matter shearing, it is very likely that the right hemisphere will appear to be more impaired than the left. This is, in one very important sense, the truth; however, it is not a reflection of more damage within the right hemisphere, but rather of more functional deficit of systems subserved primarily by the right hemisphere. In this sense, the basis for the exhibited "lateralized" deficits is functional rather than strictly physiological.

3. Children who exhibit the NLD syndrome and hence appear to be suffering from impairment of right-hemisphere systems are very likely to "rush in where angels fear to tread," including out from between parked cars and into roadways filled with speeding vehicles. Similarly, they are more prone to falling from swings, slides, bicycles, and so on than are children who are developing their psychomotor and visual-spatial-organizational skills at a normal rate. In other words, as suggested in connection with the discussion of head injury earlier in this chapter, it may be the case that many children who appear to be suffering from right-hemisphere damage *following* significant craniocerebral trauma were actually suffering from it *prior to* the trauma.

Does a Wechsler HV–LP Deviation of Significant Proportions Signal the Presence of NLD and/or Right-Hemisphere Dysfunction?

The most frequent conceptual error made by most clinicians in neuropsychology is to consider symptoms and signs of disturbance in isolation from the context of the results of a comprehensive neuropsychological evaluation. This is particularly counterproductive in the case of NLD because one "symptom" of the disturbance, a Verbal IQ well in excess of a Performance IQ, can occur as a result of disturbances that have nothing to do with the NLD syndrome or white matter dysfunction. For example, such a discrepancy can be seen in individuals who, for one reason or another, adopt a slow-but-accurate strategy on the Wechsler Performance tests (i.e., ignore the instructions to perform as quickly as possible). It can be found in persons with lower-motor-neuron disease and other afflictions that affect dexterity but not higher cognitive functions, which may result in their obtaining very low scores on the Performance scale. The same scenario, *mutatis mutandis*, obtains for the hard-of-seeing. The list of reasons for doing poorly on the Performance scale relative to the Verbal scale could go on and on. The important thing to bear in mind with respect to the analysis of the NLD syndrome is that all or virtually all of its elements should be present if the dynamics of the disturbance are to be clarified and if forms of treatment that have been shown to be suitable for the syndrome are to be instituted.

Why Is "Verbal" or "Insight-Oriented" Dynamic Psychotherapy Ineffective with the NLD Person?

Most frequently, adults exhibiting the NLD syndrome are thought to be very good candidates for verbal, insight-oriented psychotherapy. They may present with apparently well-developed verbal skills and advanced education credentials. Their symptomatology may appear to be confined to mild or moderate chronic depression, social isolation, and difficulties in obtaining and maintaining gainful employment. It is thus easy to leap to the conclusion that some degree of intrapsychic conflict is interfering with adaptation, making psychotherapy aimed at achieving insight regarding the basis of this conflict seem reasonable. Many experienced practitioners would assume that such therapy would be instrumental in the eventual lifting of the patient's depression and isolation and would allow for the marshaling of resources to maintain employment and build up fruitful interpersonal relationships.

What usually ensues when such a course of therapy is mounted, however, is that the patient appears not to achieve any insight. Rather, the same stories are told over and over again, the monotonous repetition of events appears endless, and enormous countertransference develops in the therapist. It is usually at this point that the neuropsychologist gets a chance to see the patient.

The situation that is transpiring in this instance is one more manifestation of the problems faced by persons with NLD. Because of their superficially well-developed verbal skills and the fact that they are voracious readers, they are assumed to be much more "intelligent" than really happens to be the case. It is not readily apparent, even to the fairly experienced observer, that the excessive verbiage of the patient is largely free of conceptual content and that the pragmatic aspects of these utterances are at an almost primitive level. Having "covered up" their inadequacies for years by filling the air with sound, individuals with NLD are especially prone to do so when facing the anxiety engendered by psychological assessment and the introduction of psychotherapy. (See Chapter 7 for a consideration of more preferred modes of treatment for NLD individuals.)

A FINAL NOTE

It is important to appreciate the unfolding of the NLD syndrome within the context of the investigative effort that gave birth to it. Elements of it began to be apparent in the early 1970s, with investigations involving groups of learning-disabled children differentiated on the basis of VIQ–PIQ discrepancies. Its features became clearer as we continued with validity studies aimed at determining the patterns of neuropsychological abilities and deficits of groups of learning-disabled children chosen on the basis of patterns of academic performance. Most characteristics were well known by the time we began in earnest the investigation of the concurrent and long-range socioemotional/adaptational implications of the syndrome. With the formulation of the NLD model, we are now focusing on the investigation of the manifestations of NLD in persons suffering from various forms of neurological disease, disorder, and/or dysfunction. In all of this, the clear aim has been to develop and refine a comprehensive theoretical model of brain–behavior relationships that would be capable of encompassing the life-span developmental and adaptive dimensions of learning abilities and disabilities, in all of their complex manifestations.

In the next chapter we turn to a more focused consideration of the clinical implications of the NLD syndrome and model, with regard to assessment and intervention.

CHAPTER SEVEN

Clinical Aspects of the NLD Syndrome and Model

This chapter begins with a few brief remarks pertaining to comprehensive neuropsychological assessment procedures. This is followed by a fairly extensive analysis of one clinical problem with which many NLD adolescents and adults often grapple, namely, depression and suicide risk. The bulk of the chapter is taken up with specific case illustrations of persons who exhibit the NLD syndrome and the explication of a program of general treatment recommendations that we have found to be effective for them. It is hoped that this combination of presentations will add some clinical flesh to the skeleton of the NLD syndrome and model, which were presented in the last two chapters.

NEUROPSYCHOLOGICAL ASSESSMENT PROCEDURES: CONTENT AND RATIONALE

Extensive discussions of the neuropsychological assessment procedures that we have found useful with children and adolescents can be found in Rourke (1976a, 1981), Rourke, Bakker, et al. (1983, especially Chapter 5), and Rourke, Fisk, and Strang (1986, especially Chapters 1 and 2). Only a few general points will be emphasized here.

Comprehensiveness

If a neuropsychological assessment of a child who is suspected or known to be suffering from brain disease is felt necessary, it should be comprehensive in nature. Our experience with procedures that aim simply to "screen" for brain impairment is that they typically do more harm than good. Even disregarding, for the moment, the very high levels of false positives and negatives that such procedures typically generate, it should be pointed out that it is rarely if ever useful to know simply that a child's brain is or is not impaired. In fact, such knowledge, especially when a positive "diagnosis" of brain damage is made on the basis of such an assessment procedure, may very well be counterproductive for the child. This is so because there is a very persistent myth about brain damage, which holds that brain-damaged youngsters are not amenable to therapy or intervention, and this error persists in the minds of many otherwise prudent and thoughtful caregivers. Of course, nothing could be further from the truth.

In addition, as should become apparent as we delve into the case illustrations and treatment recommendations presented later in this chapter, it is usually essential to know at least as much about what a brain-impaired child *can* do as it is to know what he or she *cannot* do, if one's goal is to design an appropriate treatment/intervention plan for the youngster. Such plans usually involve a combination of direct "attack" on the deficits and the exploitation of the child's assets for compensatory modes of adaptation. In general, the older and the more impaired the child, the more likely it is that compensatory techniques accentuating the use of the child's assets will be found effective and will tend to dominate the treatment picture. Comprehensive neuropsychological assessment procedures are designed with this "accentuate the positive" rule in mind.

But, what constitutes a comprehensive assessment? As explained in detail in the works just cited, a comprehensive neuropsychological assessment is one that involves the measurement of the principal skills and abilities that are thought to be subserved by the brain. Thus, a fairly broad sampling of tasks involving sensory, perceptual, motor/psychomotor, attentional, mnestic, linguistic, concept-formation, problem-solving, and hypothesis-testing skills would need to be administered. In addition, it would be well to vary the levels of complexity of such tasks, from quite simple to quite complex, and to present tasks that vary along the dimensions of rote versus novel requirements and information processing within a single modality versus coordination and execution of response requirements within several modalities. It is clear that these continua of tests and measures are not mutually exclusive. Finally, it is particularly important in the analysis of the NLD syndrome to have available fairly comprehensive personality and "behavioral" data on the child. Standardized tests of important dimensions of psychopathology, activity level, and common problem behaviors are quite essential for this purpose.

A collection of tests and measures that includes these dimensions would meet the minimal requirements for comprehensiveness. For a list of the tests that fulfil such criteria and that we use routinely in our evaluation of children referred for neuropsychological assessment, see the appendix to this book.

Standardized Administration Procedures and the Availability of Norms

We have found that testing procedures that are standardized and that have norms available for them are quite essential in the study of children who exhibit NLD and any number of other neuropsychological difficulties. This is so for a variety of reasons, not the least of which is the fact that the manifestations of NLD change in predictable ways over time, and this predictability is best couched in terms of deviations from age-expected performance that either declines, remains stable, or increases over time. Without the availability of developmental norms and their crucially important partners, standardized tests, it would not have been possible to isolate the NLD syndrome in the first place. Furthermore, the use of unstandardized procedures would make it all but impossible to assess the fulminations, responses to therapy, and other aspects of the syndrome's course in the individual patient. In the last analysis, standardized assessment procedures and their attendant benefits are what makes it possible to translate clinical lore into rigorous, testable clinical generalizations (e.g., the NLD syndrome and model).

Procedures Amenable to a Variety of Methods of Inference

The methods of inference for comprehensive neuropsychological assessment procedures first proposed by Reitan (1966) are as important now as they were when he articulated them. It is quite crucial (1) to be able to apply *level-of-performance* interpretations, especially within the context of developmental norms; (2) to have a sufficiently broad sample of performance so that *pathognomonic signs* of brain impairment may emerge; (3) to have data in a variety of realms that are amenable to the *differential score* approach; and (4) to be able to carry out systematic *comparisons of performance on the two sides of the body*.

In the analysis of the NLD syndrome, all of these methods of inference are employed, as the case illustrations included later in this chapter should exemplify.

There are a number of other features of comprehensive, systematic neuropsychological assessment that are important considerations in the analysis of the NLD child's behavior. These will arise in our discussion of the case illustrations that follow. More comprehensive treatments of such issues are contained in Rourke, Bakker, et al. (1983) and Rourke, Fisk, and Strang (1986).

EXAMPLE: RISK FOR DEPRESSION AND SUICIDE

We begin the illustrations of the clinical dimensions of the NLD syndrome with a discussion of a particular set of socioemotional/adaptational difficulties that is, unfortunately, faced by many adolescents and adults who exhibit the syndrome. (This presentation is adapted from a fuller account that is published in Rourke, Young, & Leenaars, 1989.) My colleagues and I have found that NLD adolescents and adults are very much at risk for progressively worsening forms of internalized psychopathology that often have suicidal behavior as one of their correlates. Of course, this is not meant to imply that other subtypes of learning-disabled children may not exhibit this type of psychopathology; however, our own research and that of others would suggest strongly that learning-disabled children whose problems in learning appear to stem from deficits in psycholinguistic skill development are less likely, on average, to exhibit this particular type of socioemotional difficulty (see Chapter 3). At this point, it would be instructive to examine briefly some of the dynamics of NLD children, adolescents, and adults that tend to promote this particular set of socioemotional difficulties.

Relevant Adaptational Difficulties
of Children and Adolescents

Psychomotor Clumsiness and Problems
in Tactile Sensitivity

The importance of psychomotor coordination and basic sensory-perceptual competencies (such as tactile sensitivity) are characteristically undervalued in most psychosocial treatments of adolescent and adult competencies. This is, of course, due primarily to the overwhelming emphasis and rather obvious importance that is accorded linguistic proficiencies in connection with adult competency and adaptation. Although not for a moment denying the value of linguistic competence for mature adaptation, it must also be pointed out that adult interactions, especially of the intimate variety, are largely functions of smooth, coordinated, integrated sensorimotor functioning and spontaneous adaptive alterations to meet sometimes rapidly changing social circumstances. These processes involve not only sensorimotor integrity but also a number of other "nonverbal" dimensions that have been discussed in connection with the NLD syndrome. Persons who are incapable of deploying such behaviors are seldom, if ever, "popular" with their peers. Indeed, they are often viewed as social misfits. The serious clinical ramifications of this state of affairs would be expected to include an increase in the probability of social withdrawal, social isolation, and depression.

Visual-Spatial-Organizational Deficits

Standing too close or too far away from other persons while engaged in various forms of social interaction; failure to appreciate subtle and sometimes even obvious visual details in configurations, with consequent misinterpretation of them; extreme difficulties in appreciating others' nonverbal "body language"; and poor appreciation of visual-spatial relationships when locomoting, driving a car, and engaging in gestures of affection are all examples of the predictable ramifications of deficits in visual-spatial-organizational skills. In addition to encouraging social ostracism for NLD children or adolescents (with unfortunate consequences such as an increase in the likelihood of withdrawal, isolation, and depression), it should also be clear that these disabilities render such persons at risk for personal injury, at the hands of others or through their own misperception and mismanagement of physical dangers. Their tendency to "rush in where angels fear to tread" is not a reflection of their courage, but rather of their failure to appreciate the dangers inherent in the situation and the consequences of their actions within it.

Difficulties in Dealing with Novelty

NLD children and adolescents have particular difficulty in adapting to situations that require systematic orientation to and analysis of novel stimulus material. This is especially the case when there exist no over-learned descriptive systems and/or patterns of adaptation for coping with them. Instead of orienting successfully to such novel situations, planning and executing adequate coping strategies, and dealing flexibly with changing patterns of interaction within them, it is quite probable that NLD children or adolescents will attempt to apply previously over-learned strategies to such situations in a stereotyped, rigid fashion. It goes without saying that such inflexible approaches are likely to meet with considerable resistance from others involved in the interaction. The predicament becomes even worse when, as is very likely to be the case, these persons attempt to deal with such situations in a verbal fashion, although some other mode of interaction (e.g., touching, psychomotor expression, appropriate gesturing) is demanded. As the inevitable social rebuffs that they experience are multiplied many times over, it is reasonable to expect that they will become prone to withdraw from such contacts after brief encounters with them. Indeed, they may eventually become seriously isolated and avoid social encounters almost entirely. Thus, we see another developmental manifestation of the NLD syndrome that would be expected, under a wide variety of circumstances, to lead directly to marked isolation and withdrawal from social intercourse, with consequent increases in the likelihood of depression.

Problems in Intermodal Integration

Included among the difficulties that arise from limitations in the capacity for intermodal integration are the following: problems in the assessment of another's emotional state through the integration of information gleaned from facial expressions, tone of voice, posture, psychomotor patterns, and so on; limitations in the assessment of social cause-and-effect relationships because of a failure to integrate data from a number of sources, which is often necessary in order to generate reasonable hypotheses regarding the chain of events in social intercourse; failure to appreciate humor because of the complex intermodal judgments required for assessing the juxtaposition of the incongruous; and imputing of unreasonable, trite, and/or oversimplified causes for the behavior of others, and imparting such assignations in situations that would lead to embarrassment for the person so described. These are but a few of the consequences that accrue for NLD children or adolescents because of the difficulties that they experience in integrating information from a variety of sources. Such unfortunate outcomes, of course, are much worse when they are anxious and confused in novel or otherwise complex situations, as becomes increasingly common with age. It should be clear that such experiences, common as they are for NLD persons, encourage withdrawal and eventual isolation from social intercourse, again with consequences vis-à-vis depression.

Consequences for Adults

The practical, concrete ramifications of the NLD syndrome in adult life are easy to understand. NLD adults typically find that their efforts to pursue their chosen professions (i.e., those for which they were educated) must be forsaken for "less demanding" jobs; and that these second-choice jobs often require smooth psychomotor coordination, trouble-shooting, and dealing adaptively with the demands of new or otherwise complex situations. They further exhibit a virtual inability to reflect on the nature and seriousness of their problems (anosognosia), as well as extreme difficulties in generating adequate solutions for those problems that they do appreciate. They also show marked deficiencies in the appreciation of subtle and even fairly obvious nonverbal aspects of communication, with consequent social disdain and even rejection.

It should be clear that this state of affairs, developing as it does over a period of years, would increase greatly the probability that those individuals so afflicted will feel that others do not wish to be with them, that their behavioral expressions are seen as silly and the object of ridicule, and that they are impotent in the face of what are for them challenging circumstances, but with which others seemingly deal without difficulty. Thus, it should come as no surprise that depression and suicide attempts are greater than average in individuals who exhibit this syndrome (Rourke, Young, et al., 1986).

Despite the damaging effects of their early experiences, many of these individuals manage to complete secondary school and move on to obtain college or university degrees. It is likely that the structure inherent in the academic milieu increases the probability that they will be able to cope and even succeed within its confines, especially if courses in mathematics, science, and similar subjects can be avoided. The most serious crises seem to occur at the point when they leave school and attempt to enter the competitive workforce. It is at this juncture that they begin to experience the most devastating effects of their deficits. Attempting to find work in line with their academic achievement, they seldom get past the interview stage, primarily because of their social ineptitude. Should they manage to obtain work, they typically fail because jobs that are seen as commensurate with their level of scholastic attainment are too complex for them. Lacking insight into this, they may continue to look for similar jobs; however, they eventually opt for less demanding work. Even then, failure is common.

Case Illustration

Some of the implications of this state of affairs are contained in the following case illustration. Some aspects of this case have been described previously (Rourke, Young, & Leenaars, 1989; Rourke, Young, et al., 1986).

Upon completion of secondary school, a woman whom I call H.S. initially worked as a salesperson in several department stores. Invariably, she was let go in each instance because, among other things, she made errors when using the cash register. Subsequently, she attempted a job as a keypunch operator but was dismissed from this position as well because she was slow in carrying out her responsibilities and prone to making many mistakes. Following this, she attempted several waitressing jobs. As would be expected, she found that she could not cope with the demands of such work, because she often got orders mixed up and her motor coordination problems made it difficult for her to carry trays, particularly during busy times when speed was demanded.

Discouraged, depressed, and by now criticized by her high-achieving, upper-class relatives, H.S. sought help from a psychologist. On the basis of a vocational assessment the psychologist advised that her interests were clearly in the "helping" professions. Following the advice of the psychologist, she subsequently managed to gain acceptance into a social work program at a university. Despite extreme difficulty, particularly in the third and fourth years when the academic and practical (field placement) demands became quite complex, she managed to complete the program. This was accomplished, however, only with considerable help from others in organizing term papers, in writing reports, and in other aspects of the academic program. She also received much in the way of general support from a sympathetic guidance counselor.

During this 4-year period, H.S. experienced bouts of severe anxiety and depression; however, it was not until after her graduation and subsequent futile job searches that her suicide attempts began. Over a period of 2 years, she "overdosed" three times and was admitted to a psychiatric unit on each occasion. Misunderstood by her relatives, who continued to demand that she should be working "like everyone else"; out of touch with her former school friends because they were all either busy working or raising children; rejected by potential employers; and incapable of comprehending the nature and implications of her deficits, she finally (and very reluctantly) assented to receiving a disability pension. With considerable supportive counseling, she has not attempted suicide for several years, but she is chronically depressed and frequently talks about being "no good" and of "no use to anyone."

H.S. continues to believe that she could function as a social worker if she could only obtain such a position. In all likelihood, she could never do so. While she possesses a rudimentary knowledge of the field, she lacks the cognitive capacity to evaluate complex situations adequately, the cognitive/affective flexibility to deal with the changing needs of individual clients, and the emotional strength to survive the stresses inherent in even a light caseload. She is highly vulnerable to stress and, as an apparent result of this, has developed multiple physical symptoms over the years. As well, she endured a period of approximately 6 months during which she was clearly paranoid, with delusions mainly of persecution. She is currently functioning reasonably well, but it is clear that even the prospect of maintaining a small apartment, preparing meals for herself, and coping with the other requirements of daily living represent a considerable challenge for her.

Interestingly, H.S. has, on several occasions, expressed a desire to apply to graduate school to obtain an M.A. in social work, convinced that this would be the "ticket" to her success. Thus, her unrealistic self-evaluation is perpetuated in the belief that another degree will solve the problem. In fact, in the unlikely event that she could complete a graduate program, the stage would be set for new and even more devastating setbacks.

Conclusions

Suicide is probably best understood as a multidimensional malaise (Shneidman, 1985). It would seem most accurate to define it as an event with biological (including biochemical), sociocultural, interpersonal, psychological, and personal philosophical/existential aspects. It is also possible to attempt to structure suicidal phenomena from a neuropsychological point of view, a perspective that is often neglected in reviews related to the biology of suicide (see Maris, 1986). Specifically, the following question arises: Why does the person who exhibits the NLD syndrome appear to have a higher incidence of suicidal behavior than do (1) persons who exhibit different learning disability subtypes and (2) persons with well-documented brain damage who do not exhibit this syndrome?

A review of the literature on suicide and neuropsychology, including the literature on learning disabilities, resulted in only a few citations of works pertaining to this issue (i.e., Casey, 1977; Kenny, Rohn, Sarles, Reynolds, & Heald, 1979; Peck, 1985; Robins, West, & Murphy, 1977; Rohn, Sarles, Kenny, Reynolds, & Heald, 1977; Simpson, 1975; Smith, 1982). One consistent and important observation in this literature is that persons with a diagnosed learning disability or demonstrable brain injury are thought to be in an "at risk" group. For example, Peck (1985) asserted the following association between suicide and learning disabilities: "It is clear that learning disabled youngsters may suffer from loss of esteem, and in those cases where the youngsters experienced both pressure from parents to be 'normal' and pressure from peers regarding their disability, their feelings of frustration and hurt may be so great as to place a very young child in an at risk category for suicide" (p. 116).

Although Peck's (1985) observations are important for understanding the development of suicidal behavior, he does not take note of the view that particular subtypes of learning disability may render a person at risk for socioemotional pathology, whereas other subtypes of learning disability do not appear to have the same proclivity (see Chapter 3). The contention in the current discussion is that persons manifesting the NLD syndrome are particularly at risk for socioemotional disturbance of the internalized variety and, in turn, for suicide.

Suicide in adolescents and adults has been related to a variety of phenomena, including the following: (1) unemployment, job loss, school and professional failure, and other career coping problems (Barnes, 1986; Hendin, 1985; Leenaars, in press; Maris, 1985; Shneidman, 1985); (2) inability to cope or solve problems in general (Leenaars, Balance, Wenckstern, & Rudzinski, 1985; Menninger, 1938; Peck, 1985; Shneidman, 1985); and (3) marked interpersonal conflict and especially rejection

(Freud 1920/1974; Leenaars, 1988; Leenaars et al., 1985; Murray, 1967; Shneidman, 1985). The similarity between these descriptors and the characteristics, manifestations, and consequences of the NLD syndrome are obvious, as illustrated by the case of H.S. Withdrawal, anxiety, and depression have also been well documented in both the NLD syndrome and in those thought to be at particular risk for suicide. This confluence of events for persons exhibiting the NLD syndrome—that is, repeated failures in coping, combined with loss of esteem, feelings of inferiority, emotional confusion and distress, and any number of other socioemotional/adaptational strains within the personality—constitutes an "at risk" state for suicide. Furthermore, it should be clear that those who exhibit this syndrome are at risk for many forms of internalized psychopathology, whether or not they actually participate in suicidal behavior (see Chapters 4 and 5).

In this section it has been emphasized that the NLD syndrome appears to predispose those so afflicted to suicide risk. This is not meant to suggest that all persons who exhibit the NLD syndrome are suicidal. The point is that, since suicide is a multidimensional event, the NLD component in addition to other biological, sociocultural, and interpersonal components in a needful individual may result in that individual defining an issue for which suicide is perceived as the best solution. As suggested in Chapters 5 and 6, this syndrome is manifest in many types of neurological disease/dysfunction, the risk for a variety of forms of internalized psychopathology is high in such individuals, and the manifestations of the syndrome are best thought of as indications of learning disability. There is no intended implication here that children whose learning disabilities appear to stem from deficits in psycholinguistic skill development may not manifest socioemotional disturbance, or that they may not be at greater-than-normal risk for suicidal behavior. Rather, it is suggested that such manifestations are significantly and markedly greater in NLD children, adolescents, and adults than in persons exhibiting other subtypes of learning disability, and that these manifestations are predictable adaptive outcomes of the particular pattern of neuropsychological abilities and deficits that constitutes the NLD syndrome.

BACKGROUND FOR CASE PRESENTATIONS

We turn now to the presentation of a series of case illustrations of children and adolescents who exhibit the NLD syndrome. These cases were chosen with a view to highlighting the principal features and dynamics of the syndrome. Although some specific treatment recommendations are mentioned periodically within these cases, reference to the section toward the end of this chapter is necessary in order to appreciate the general outlines of the treatment program that we have found to be most effective with such youngsters.

To facilitate discussion, each of the five case presentations has been assigned a gender-appropriate pseudonym. The general format for the presentations involves an introduction containing some information regarding the patient, a presentation of the neuropsychological test results, and a discussion of the findings. The test results are arranged in a manner that is meant to facilitate their interpretation within the context of the NLD syndrome. The tests employed in this battery are described in the appendix and are discussed at length in Rourke, Bakker, et al. (1983) and Rourke, Fisk, and Strang (1986). For the most part, the neuropsychological test results are couched in terms of the sets of characteristics that describe the NLD syndrome. Some notes regarding the format of data presentation are in order, as follows:

1. In these case descriptions, the terms *severe, moderate, mild, borderline, average,* and *superior* are used to describe levels of impairment on tests within the various areas discussed. On the basis of the Knights and Norwood (1980) norms for these tests, these terms indicate the following levels of impairment: (a) *severe* means more than 3 SDs below the mean for the age of the child; (b) *moderate* means between 2 and 3 SDs below the mean; (c) *mild* means between 1 and 2 SDs below the mean; and (d) *borderline* means close to 1 SD below the mean. *Average* means between 1 SD below and 1 SD above the mean, and *superior* means performance that exceeds 1 SD above the mean.

2. A range of *T* scores from 10 to 60 is used throughout. Those scores that fall below 10 and above 60 are assigned scores of 10 and 60, respectively. This poses a significant problem only for scores that are considerably higher than 60; these are pointed out in the text account of the assessment.

3. To facilitate interpretation, the WISC and WISC-R summary measures, and (when available) the results for the Personality Inventory for Children (PIC), the Activity Rating Sacle (ARS), the Behavior Problem Checklist (BPC), and the Vineland Adaptive Behavior Scale

(VABS; Sparrow, Balla, & Cicchetti, 1984) are presented in numerical format.

4. Because of the nature of the qualitative analysis of responses on the Aphasia Screening Test, these results are presented in textual, rather than graphical, form. Other dimensions of qualitative analysis are also presented in the text.

CASE 1: MARY[1]

This case is presented in order to illustrate the clinical manifestations of the NLD syndrome in a child with significant white matter disease involving absence of the commissural fibers.

Note on Presentation. This first case presentation is especially detailed. This was thought to be advisable so that the reader would be able to examine in detail the manifestations and dynamics of the NLD syndrome. Subsequent case illustrations are somewhat briefer and have different emphases.

Relevant History

A CT scan was interpreted as reflecting virtually complete agenesis of the corpus callosum. The CT scan was carried out as part of a neurological work-up of Mary because she was afflicted with a seizure disorder. At the time of testing, she was on a regimen of anticonvulsant medication (1000 mg Depakene per day and 200 mg Tegretol 3 times daily); her last seizure had occurred approximately 4 months prior to the neuropsychological examination. She was referred for assessment primarily because of problems in academic performance (she experienced difficulty in "producing" on tests and in situations where speed and adaptability of response were required) and because of what were thought to be accompanying socioemotional deviations. Mary underwent two comprehensive neuropsychological assessments; one at 9 years and one at 11½ years of age. The WISC and the WRAT were administered in the first examination; the WISC-R and the WRAT-R, in the second assessment. Otherwise, the same tests were administered in

---

[1]Aspects of this case have been presented previously, in Rourke (1987).

both examinations. These results are summarized graphically in Figure 7.1.[2]

The main points of the following description deal with the findings of the initial assessment at 9 years of age. This is followed by a brief summary of the major findings of the second assessment, including an analysis of the results of the VABS which was administered at that time. It should be noted that there was virtually no change in Mary's pattern of neuropsychological test results from the first to the second assessment; however, there were some changes evident in her pattern of scores on the measures of personality, activity level, and behavioral problems at the time of the second examination.

First Assessment

Tactile perception. There were no indications of any simple tactile imperception with either hand. Mary exhibited moderate tactile suppression with the left hand; there were no indications of tactile suppression with the right hand. Her levels of performance were moderately to severely impaired with both hands on tests for finger agnosia, finger

---

[2]Explanation of abbreviations used in figures: *Tactile*: TAC-R, tactile-perceptual abilities, right hand; TAC-L, tactile-perceptual abilities, left hand; FNA-R, finger agnosia, right hand; FNA-L, finger agnosia, left hand; FTWR-R, fingertip number-writing, right hand; FTWR-L, fingertip number-writing, left hand; TACF-R, tactile–forms recognition, right hand; TACF-L, tactile–forms recognition, left hand. *Motor & Psychomotor*: DYN-R, dynamometer (strength of grip), right hand; DYN-L, dynamometer (strength of grip), left hand; FiT-R, finger tapping, right hand; FiT-L, finger tapping, left hand; HOL-RT, Graduated Holes Test, time, right hand; HOL-RC, Graduated Holes Test, contact, right hand; HOL-LT, Graduated Holes Test, time, left hand; HOL-LC, Graduated Holes Test, contact, left hand; FoT-R, foot tapping, right foot, FoT-L, foot tapping, left foot; MZ-RT, Maze Test, time, right hand; MZ-RC, Maze Test, contact, right hand; MZ-LT, Maze Test, time, left hand; MZ-LC, Maze Test, contact, left hand; PEG-R, Grooved Pegboard, right hand; PEG-L, Grooved Pegboard, left hand. *Visual-Spatial*: PICCOM, WISC Picture Completion; PICTAR, WISC Picture Arrangement; BLOCDE, WISC Block Design; OBJASS, WISC Object Assembly; TARGET, Target Test. *Verbal*: PPVT, Peabody Picture Vocabulary Test; INFO, WISC Information; COMP, WISC Comprehension; ARITH, WISC Arithmetic; SIMIL, WISC Similarities; VOCAB, WISC Vocabulary; DIGITS, WISC Digit Span; SSPER, Speech-Sounds Perception Test; AUDCLO, Auditory Closure Test; SENMEM, Sentence Memory Test; FLUENCY, Verbal Fluency Test. *Problem Solving, Etc.*: CODING, WISC Coding; TMT-A, Trail Making Test, Part A; TMT-B, Trail Making Test, Part B; TPT-Dom, Tactual Performance Test, dominant hand; TPT-ND, Tactual Performance Test, nondominant hand; TPT-Bo, Tactual Performance Test, both hands, TPT-Tot, Tactual Performance Test, total; TPT-Mem, Tactual Performance Test, memory; TPT-Loc, Tactual Performance Test, location; Cat-T, Category Test.

dysgraphesthesia, and astereognosis for coins. Her tactile perceptual problems were somewhat more marked with the left hand on the test for finger agnosia.

Motor and psychomotor skills. Mary was almost exclusively left-handed, right-footed, and left-eyed. She exhibited moderate to severe bilateral deficiencies in grip strength, finger- and foot-tapping speed, and psychomotor coordination under speeded conditions (Grooved Pegboard Test). She also experienced difficulties with the left hand on the Holes Test for static tremor, and mild to moderate deficiencies with the left hand on the Maze Coordination Test for kinetic tremor. She performed at a severely impaired level on the Speed subtest of the Underlining Test, which requires speeded performance in the absence of virtually any requirement for visual discrimination. In general, her motoric deficiencies were somewhat more marked with the left hand, especially when hand dominance was taken into consideration (note her left- versus right-hand performance on the Finger Tapping and Maze Tests as shown in Figure 7.1). Her levels of performance with each hand separately and with both hands together on the Tactual Performance Test were severely impaired. On the latter test, performance was especially impaired with the left (dominant) hand: Mary placed only three of the six blocks correctly before the left-hand trial was terminated at 15 minutes.

Visual-spatial-organizational abilities. On the Performance section of the WISC, she obtained outstandingly low scaled scores on the Picture Arrangement and Object Assembly subtests. Her level of performance on the Target Test, designed as a measure of immediate memory for visual sequences, approached the moderately impaired level. She had mild difficulties with the Trail Making Test. Much of her performance on the Underlining Test was quite poor: She performed at mildly to severely impaired levels on 8 of the 13 critical subtests. She exhibited considerable difficulty with cursive script, and her drawing of a complex key on the Aphasia Screening Test was quite immature and lacking in visual-spatial detail.

Rote memory. Mary obtained scaled scores ranging from 10 to 13 on the Information, Vocabulary, and Digit Span subtests of the WISC. Her performance on the Sentence Memory Test was at a borderline level. Memory for this sort of material contrasted rather sharply with her levels of performance on other tests requiring more effortful processing, such as the Target Test and the last subtest of the Category Test.

Speech and language characteristics. Mary's misspellings (Aphasia Screening Test, WRAT) were almost exclusively of the phonetically

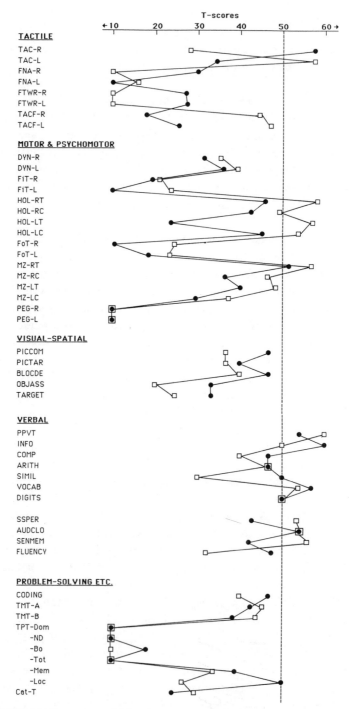

FIGURE 7.1. Summary of Mary's neuropsychological test results. ●——●, first testing; □——□, second testing.

154

	Testing 1 (9 yr, 0 mo)	Testing 2 (11 yr, 6 mo)
WISC[a]		
VIQ	104	88
PIQ	85	70
FSIQ	94	78
Underlining (no. of each)		
Superior	0	0
Average	2	2
Borderline	3	4
Mild	2	0
Moderate	4	6
Severe	2	1
Speed subtest (impairment)	Severe	Moderate
WRAT[b] (grade; centile)		
Reading	6.9; 91	8; 87
Spelling	6.5; 92	8; 94
Arithmetic	4.1; 55	4; 16
PIC (T score)		
Lie	34	38
F	96	96
Defensiveness	43	35
Adjustment	69	83
Achievement	43	54
Intellectual Screening	99	120
Development	49	73
Somatic Concern	92	89
Depression	78	79
Family Relations	45	45
Delinquency	58	64
Withdrawal	62	62
Anxiety	71	68
Psychosis	97	93
Hyperactivity	73	57
Social Skills	86	93
ARS		
No	1	0
Little	16	25
Very much	15	7
BPC		
No	11	18
Little	25	40
Very much	28	7

	Standard score	Centile	Age-equivalent score
VABS (at 11½ yr only)			
Communication	64	1	7 yr, 5 mo
Daily Living	<20	<1	3 yr, 4 mo
Socialization	48	<1	3 yr, 6 mo
Motor		<1	2 yr, 5 mo
Adaptive Behavior Composite		<1	5 yr, 7 mo
Maladaptive Scale (raw score: 17; significant)			

[a]WISC-R, testing 2; [b]WRAT-R, testing 2.

FIGURE 7.1. (continued)

APHASIA SCREENING TEST
First examination: Mary showed no evidence of naming, reading, or auditory-verbal comprehension deficits. She had considerable difficulty in the enunciation of complex multisyllable words and made one arithmetic error ($17 \times 3 = 23$). Her misspellings were phonetically accurate. She exhibited very large, uncoordinated cursive script. There were mild visual-spatial distortions in simple drawings, as well as an extremely immature graphic rendering of a complex key. Second examination: She showed no evidence of naming or reading deficits, but there were borderline problems in auditory-verbal comprehension. She had borderline difficulty in the enunciation of multisyllabic words, made no arithmetic errors, and gave phonetically accurate misspellings. Her cursive script was fair. Mild visual-spatial distortions showed up in simple drawings, and she again gave an extremely immature graphic rendering of a complex key.

EXAMPLE FROM WRAT SPELLING SUBTEST

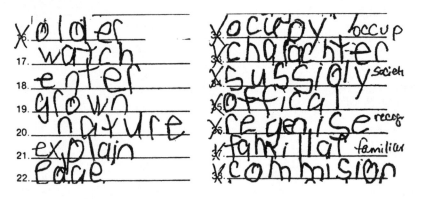

accurate variety (Sweeney & Rourke, 1978). She performed at average levels on the Peabody Picture Vocabulary Test, the Auditory Closure Test, the Speech-Sounds Perception Test, the Sentence Memory Test, and the Verbal Fluency Test. (It is very common for NLD children to perform much less well than did Mary on the Sentence Memory and Verbal Fluency Tests, probably due to the semantic and novel processing requirements of these tests.) She tended to do somewhat less well on verbal tasks that required some degree of verbal processing (e.g., the WISC Comprehension and Arithmetic subtests) than on those requiring skills of a more rote nature (e.g., the WISC Information and Vocabulary subtests). Her ambient behavior in the testing situation was marked by much verbosity and a clear tendency to seek information through verbal questioning rather than through exploration and physical experimentation.

Nonverbal problem solving, concept formation, hypothesis testing, and ability to benefit from informational feedback. Mary's level of performance on the Category Test was moderately impaired, and her overall level of timed performance on the Tactual Performance Test was severely impaired. Both of these tests require strategy generation, hypothesis testing, and problem solving under novel circumstances, and the capacity to benefit from informational feedback in such problem-solving situations. Difficulties in dealing with cause-and-effect relationships were evident on both of these tests and on the Picture Arrangement subtest of the WISC. She also exhibited an impaired level of performance on the Object Assembly subtest of the WISC. Her PIQ was 19 points below her VIQ on the WISC. Throughout the testing sessions, there was much evidence of difficulty in dealing with humor and other forms of incongruity.

Adaptation to novel, complex situations; reliance on rote behaviors. Her problems in adaptation to situations involving these dimensions were especially notable on the Category Test and on the Tactual Performance Test. In both of these testing situations, she exhibited clear evidence of perseveration and difficulties in applying problem-solving strategies to the tasks at hand in a flexible, adaptive fashion.

Reading, spelling, and arithmetic. Mary's levels of performance on the Reading (word-recognition) and Spelling subtests of the WRAT were well above average. Her level of performance on the Arithmetic subtest, although at an average level, was significantly inferior to her levels of attainment on the Reading and Spelling subtests. She obtained a WISC Arithmetic subtest scaled score of 9. On the Aphasia Screening Test she made an error on a very simple arithmetic problem. On the WRAT Arithmetic subtest she omitted details such as decimals and dollar signs from her answers, and she exhibited some perseverations in her mechanical arithmetic performance.

Social judgment, social interaction, and socioemotional functioning. As is apparent in the PIC (Wirt et al., 1977) results, which are based on her mother's responses, Mary is seen as deficient in social relations with persons outside of her immediate family, and as having a tendency toward an internalized form of psychopathology that is characterized by anxiety, social withdrawal, depression, and inappropriate interpersonal behavior. These observations were borne out in the parents' responses on the ARS and the BPC.

Second Assessment

Some features of the results of the second assessment should be noted. There were drops in Verbal, Performance, and Full Scale IQs on the WISC-R, relative to the WISC, of 16, 15, and 16 points, respectively. There were especially large declines on the Similarities and Object Assembly subtests, whereas average scores on the Information, Arithmetic, Vocabulary, and Digit Span subtests were obtained. Mary made some 2½ years of progress in the Reading and Spelling subtests of the WRAT-R; there was no evidence of advancement on the Arithmetic subtest over this period. There was worsening of finger agnosia and dysgraphesthesia, but considerably less astereognosis for coins. Her performance on all of the psychomotor measures remained in the moderately to severely impaired range, with the exception of the measures of static and kinetic steadiness. There was a decline in age-appropriate verbal fluency; in this and in some other instances, Mary's pattern of performance in this second assessment became even more typical of that expected in the NLD syndrome. Some advances were evident in cursive script, but her drawing of a key was extremely poor. Mary performed marginally better, though still at a moderately impaired level, on the Category Test. No advancement was noted on the Tactual Performance Test; in fact, there was some worsening in her level of age-appropriate performance. She exhibited marginal advances on the Trail Making Test. There were some declines in performance on aspects of the Underlining Test and the Target Test.

On the PIC there were markedly higher T scores evident on the Adjustment, Intellectual Screening, and Development scales; there was a significantly lower T score in evidence on the Hyperactivity scale. The drop on the latter was also reflected in the mother's ratings on the ARS and the BPC. (As noted in an earlier chapter, it is quite typical for children with the NLD syndrome to be rated as hyperactive at the preschool and early elementary school levels, with a gradual diminution in rated activity level to the point of hypoactivity at the early adolescent and subsequent developmental levels.) The results of the VABS are quite interesting. Note that centiles for all of the domains (Communication, Daily Living, Socialization, Motor) and the Adaptive Behavior Composite are 1 or less. This is typical for children who exhibit the NLD syndrome. Also typical of such children above the age of 9 years is the finding that the standard and age-equivalent scores for the Communication domain are significantly higher (although markedly impaired relative to age norms) than are their respective scores for the other domains.

The Maladaptive Scale score of 17 is quite "significant" with respect to the amount of socioemotional deviation evident in this child.

Discussion: NLD Elements and Dynamics

It should be clear from the preceding description that Mary's profile of neuropsychological abilities and deficits fits the clinical features of the NLD syndrome rather well. There are some deviations from this pattern, however, which will be discussed. It should be borne in mind that Mary's academic placement at the time of the second assessment was in a "general learning disabilities" class, which is usually reserved for children of Mary's age who are thought to be functioning at the mildly retarded to low borderline level of intelligence. She had been placed in this educational setting because school officials felt strongly that her general and specific levels of adaptive functioning were certainly no better than those of her classmates. Indeed, they felt that, in the main, her adaptive skills were significantly poorer than the general class level.

A consideration of the elements and dynamics of the NLD syndrome in this case would be instructive. This account stresses the changes in evidence between the first and second evaluations. (Remember that the WISC and WRAT were administered in the first examination and the WISC-R and WRAT-R in the second. In the text, the differences in difficulty levels of these instruments are taken into consideration.) In the following, assets are coded (A) and listed first, followed by deficits, coded (D).

Simple motor skills. (A) and (D): Although there were some "advances" in evidence, Mary's simple motor skills (grip strength, finger tapping) remained, for the most part, moderately to severely impaired over the 2½ year period examined. However, there were significant improvements in static tremor in evidence on the Holes Test.

Complex psychomotor skills. (A): There was some evidence of gains on the Mazes Test of kinetic tremor. (D): In both testings, there were marked difficulties bilaterally in foot tapping speed and on tests involving complex psychomotor skills (Grooved Pegboard Test; Tactual Performance Test). There was outstandingly poor performance on the Motor domain of the VABS.

Tactile perception. (A): There was no evidence of simple tactile imperception in either testing, and there was considerable lessening of astereognosis for coins at the second testing. (D): Moderate to severe degrees of tactile suppression (left hand) and other tactile-perceptual deficiencies were found in both testings. There was some evidence of a preponderance of errors on the left side in the first testing.

Visual perception. (D): Poor scores were obtained on all of the Wechsler Performance subtests at the second testing, as well as extreme difficulties on WISC-R Object Assembly subtest. Visual-spatial distortions and difficulties in dealing with complex detail were noted in Mary's graphic rendering of visual designs during both assessments. Very poor scores on the Underlining Test, especially for subtests involving visually complex target items, were prominent in both examinations.

Auditory perception. (A): An advance in performance was in evidence on the Speech-Sounds Perception Test; performance on the Auditory Closure Test remained relatively stable. Phonetically accurate misspellings were prominent in both examinations.

Rote material. (A): Advances were in evidence in cursive script. Age-appropriate progress was noted in reading and spelling. Digit Span scores remained age-appropriate in the second examination.

Novel material. (D): There was markedly impaired performance on the Category Test and the Tactual Performance Test over time. WISC and WISC-R Performance subtests were dealt with in a poor fashion in both testings, with some evidence of decline at the time of the second testing with the WISC-R.

Attention. (A): Considerable progress was noted on the Seashore Rhythm Test, but performance remained at a markedly impaired level. No difficulties were found on WISC or WISC-R Digit Span or on the Auditory Closure and Speech-Sounds Perception Tests. There was evidence of considerable advancement in the matching of dictated words with their visual illustrations on the Peabody Picture Vocabulary Test. There was borderline evidence of advances in verbally guided behavior on the Trail Making Test over time. (D): Marked difficulties with the Target Test persisted over time. Attention to visual detail on the subtests of the WISC and WISC-R was moderately to severely impaired; there was some evidence of worsening in this area at the time of the second testing with the WISC-R. There was considerable evidence of impairment on both administrations of the Underlining Test; this was especially marked for complex visual material.

Exploratory behavior. (D): No evidence of curiosity regarding novel surroundings and testing equipment was apparent in the first examination, and this general avoidance of exploration persisted at the time of the second assessment.

Memory. (A): Wechsler Information, Vocabulary, and Digit Span subtests remained fairly stable over time. Sentence Memory Test performance increased over time. (D): The Memory component of the Tactual Performance Test was poor in both testings, and there was no advancement in memory at the time of the second testing, even though this was the second administration of the test and presumably was no longer a test of *incidental* memory. Target Test performance was clearly impaired in both testings. The Memory subtest of the Category Test was performed very poorly in both assessments. Almost without exception, differences between good memory for rote material and impaired memory for complex material and that which is not readily coded in a verbal fashion increased with age.

Nonverbal problem solving, concept formation, hypothesis testing, and ability to benefit from informational feedback. (D): Extreme problems on the Category Test and Tactual Performance Test (TPT) were found in both assessments. There were clear difficulties in benefiting from experience on the TPT, with negligible or no evidence of positive transfer-of-training effect found from the first to the second trial on both tests, as well as a very poor Location component in the second testing with the TPT. Problem-solving aspects of the WISC and WISC-R Performance subtests and the WRAT-R Arithmetic subtest at the time of the second testing were very poorly addressed. No clear evidence of any increases in flexible problem solving, strategy generation, or hypothesis testing were shown over time; most evidence pointed to relative declines in these areas.

Speech and language. (A): Misspellings were almost exclusively of the phonetically accurate variety. There was no evidence of impairment on the Auditory Closure Test, and there was a significant gain on the Speech-Sounds Perception Test. Much better than age-appropriate gains were made between the two examinations on the Peabody Picture Vocabulary Test. Wechsler Information and Vocabulary subtests remained at normal levels. There was much verbosity in both testings and no frankly aphasic signs in either assessment. (D): Mildly deficient oral-motor praxis was shown in both examinations. There was no appreciable speech prosody, and a high volume of verbal output was found. Errors on the Sentence Memory Test were almost exclusively of the phonological variety in both examinations. There was poor quality of content and pragmatics in verbal utterances. Preference was shown for "exploration" of the environment by verbal rather than psychomotor means. Mary had marked difficulties in the generating of words to a rule (Verbal Fluency Test), in spite of a high volume of verbal output. Although the highest score obtained on the VABS, the Communication domain score was at a severely impaired level. Deficient areas of linguistic performance showed a marked tendency to worsen with the passing of time.

Academic skills. (A): Somewhat better cursive script was found in the second assessment. Mary made age-appropriate advances on WRAT Reading and Spelling subtests, with scores at or above centile = 87 on both testings for both subtests. Verbatim memory for nonmeaningful verbal material remained good over time. (D): Arithmetic performance did not rise above the 4th-grade level at the time of the second testing. Reading comprehension was rated as very poor. The gap between reading and spelling (high) and mechanical arithmetic (low) increased over time. Courses involving problem solving and concept formation of even less than age-appropriate levels were too difficult for Mary. The gap between her extremely poor performance in subjects involving any degree of scientific reasoning and her well-developed automatic verbal skills (e.g., PPVT Mental Age of 10 years at first testing rose to 15 years, 3 months at the second testing) increased with age.

Socioemotional/adaptational skills. (D): The age-equivalent score on the Socialization domain of the VABS was 3 years, 6 months. The VABS Adaptive Behavior Composite age-equivalent score stood at 5 years, 7 months, indicating extreme deficiencies in a variety of age-appropriate adaptive skills. The PIC T score for the F scale was markedly elevated at both testings, and the overall Adjustment scale rose from 69 to 83 between the two evaluations. These scores suggest a significant level of concern on the part of her mother for Mary's general adaptational well-being, and an increased perception of indications of socioemotional disturbance over time. An increase in elevation between the two testings on the PIC Development scale reflected Mary's continuing failure to meet age-appropriate developmental demands. The elevations on the PIC Social Skills scale pointed to deep concern over Mary's capacity to comport herself in social situations. The overall clinical picture on the PIC reflected marked internalized psychopathology that was more prominent at the time of the second evaluation. The decline on the Hyperactivity scale of the PIC and the scores on the ARS and BPC were indicative of decreased levels of general activity. Taken together, the findings on the PIC, ARS, and BPC suggested a significant increase in socioemotional disturbance of the internalized variety, decreasing levels of social competence, and decreases in levels of general activity. The "significant" Maladaptive score on the VABS and the aforementioned extremely low Adaptive Behavior Composite served to reinforce this impression.

These test results were treated in detail in order to emphasize their correspondence to the general and specific features of the NLD syndrome. (Subsequent case illustrations will not reflect this degree of detailed examination.) This analysis would certainly confirm that Mary reflects the assets and deficits of the NLD syndrome rather precisely. It is also the case that the propositions of the general treatment program outlined toward the end of this chapter are quite appropriate for Mary.

CASE 2: CATHY[3]

Relevant History

This 13-year-old girl was admitted to hospital following a severe head injury that she sustained while riding a motorcycle. The following day, her pupils dilated, she became deeply comatose, and she started to decerebrate. Investigations revealed bleeding over the right cerebral hemisphere. A craniotomy was performed, which revealed severe contusions and lacerations of the right temporal and parietal lobe regions. Acute swelling of the brain necessitated excision of the entire right temporal lobe and part of the parietal lobe. The postoperative course was complicated by a respiratory obstruction requiring a tracheotomy. Otherwise, her progress was uneventful and she was discharged from hospital approximately 1 month after the latter operation. On discharge, she was able to move and walk without assistance, although a relative weakness of the left arm and leg was present. A neuropsychological assessment was requested in order to determine the residual effects of the head trauma and subsequent surgery. The first of these was carried out 5 weeks after the craniotomy was performed, and a second followed about 6 months later. The results of these tests are summarized in Figure 7.2.

Note on Relevance. From the perspective of attempting to understand the manifestations of the NLD syndrome, there are two features of the differences between Mary and Cathy that are of principal importance. The first relates to the fact that there was never a time in Mary's life when her neurological structures and systems were "normal," while Cathy experienced the benefits of some 13 years of "normal" development prior

[3]Aspects of this case have been presented previously, in Rourke, Bakker, et al. (1983), pp. 230–238.

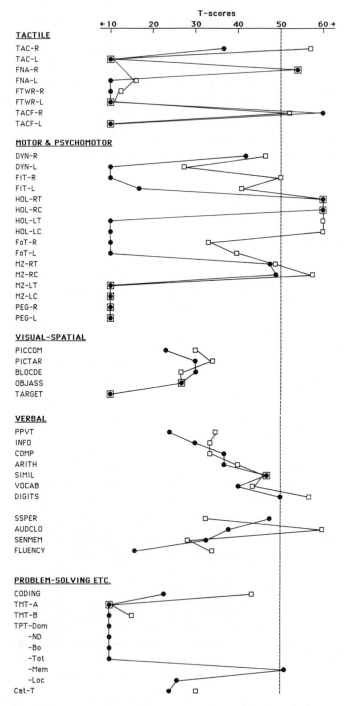

FIGURE 7.2. Summary of Cathy's neuropsychological test results. ●—●, first testing; □—□, second testing.

	Testing 1 (13 yr, 11 mo)	Testing 2 (14 yr, 5 mo)
WISC		
VIQ	81	84
PIQ	51	62
FSIQ	64	71
WRAT (grade; centile)		
Reading	6.5; 23	6.3; 16
Spelling	6.3; 21	7.4; 30
Arithmetic	2.9; 2	4.4; 4

APHASIA SCREENING TEST

First examination: Cathy encountered difficulty with items requiring her to carry out simple arithmetic computations (one oral, one written), and there was some evidence of mild problems with the enunciation of complex multisyllabic words. In addition, her drawing of a complex key was very primitive and evidence of some visual-spatial distortion was noted in her drawings, especially those of a Greek cross. Her drawings were also poorly organized on the page. Second examination: There was minor evidence of visual-spatial distortion in her drawings of a Greek cross, and her drawing of a key was again extremely primitive. Difficulty with the enunciation of complex multisyllabic words was also noted and she failed to compute one simple arithmetic problem presented orally. Otherwise, her performance was unremarkable.

EXAMPLE FROM WRAT SPELLING SUBTEST

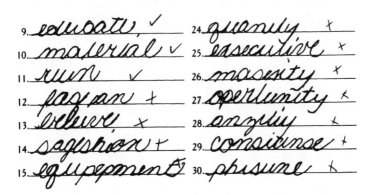

to the onset of her neurological disease. Second, the type of neuropathology from which Mary suffered is one that was chronic and long standing at the time of both of her neuropsychological assessments. This might imply that the type of cerebral organization that Mary exhibited at those times represented a series of "compromises" and "compensations" that had taken place in her cerebral neurological systems since birth, or perhaps before. Cathy, however, was tested shortly after the craniocerebral and surgical trauma suffered to her brain, and it might be inferred that no great degree of reorganization of her presumably normal premorbid cerebral systems had taken place since the time of her accident and surgery. These differences are of interest and will be addressed to some extent in the presentation of Cathy's test results. At the same time, it should be emphasized that Mary and Cathy, in spite of their vastly different developmental histories and neurological disorders, have a great deal in common in terms of patterns of neuropsychological, academic, and socioemotional functioning: Their commonality lies in their manifestations of the patterns of performance that mirror the NLD syndrome.

Behavioral Observations during the Examinations

Although possibly somewhat anxious, Cathy was reasonably friendly and seemed to try to cooperate with the examiner in the first assessment. From time to time, she appeared somewhat disoriented and confused, but the examiner was usually able to redirect her attention to the task at hand. It was frequently necessary to repeat instructions, and she seemed to interpret verbal statements in a somewhat "concrete" or literal fashion. Throughout the examination, Cathy was extremely talkative, exhibiting somewhat tangential, rambling conversation.

A second assessment was conducted approximately 6 months after the first, in order to monitor any possible changes in Cathy's adaptive ability structure. Her behavior during this second assessment was considerably more agitated than was previously noted. She was extremely distractible and very impulsive, and she became easily frustrated when unable to complete a task properly. She often seemed to become confused in the middle of a task, appearing to forget what was required of her. Throughout the examination, she was extremely loquacious, tending to "ramble on" with many complaints regarding her current academic placement and other topics.

Discussion: NLD Elements and Dynamics

There are several features of these neuropsychological test results that relate rather directly to the features of the NLD syndrome.

1. The simple tactile-perceptual deficiencies in evidence were entirely predictable, in view of the cerebral lesions and tissue extirpation that transpired in this case. The same holds true for the evidence of virtually complete left-visual-field hemianopsia (not reported in Figure 7.2). What may not be so obvious are the extremely marked deficits in visual-spatial-organizational skills that are evident in both examinations, especially on the Performance subtests of the WISC. Essentially, Cathy received credits in the latter areas for being present at the examination. It should also be noted, however, that she did not exhibit any marked constructional dyspraxia in the graphic rendering of simple visual designs; this was the case in spite of her left hemianopsia and the marked visual-spatial-organizational deficits just noted. It would appear probable that she was able to guide her constructional performance when copying from designs by directing and monitoring her behavior through verbal means. However, the much more complex demands of tasks such as the WISC Block Design and Object Assembly subtests were very much beyond her capabilities for so doing.

2. Cathy was unable to perform at anything approaching normal levels with her left hand on any of the motor and psychomotor tests. Her participation in most of these tests had to be terminated shortly after she began them because of her great difficulty. In the first assessment, it is notable that Cathy's performance on a test of simple motor skills (i.e., grip strength with the right hand) was much better, relative to age-based norms, than was her performance on a test of more complex psychomotor skills (i.e., Grooved Pegboard Test). At the time of the second assessment, this dissociation between simple motor and complex psychomotor skills was especially apparent. This pattern of *bilateral* psychomotor coordination deficiencies was exhibited in both examinations, as would be expected in persons who manifest the NLD syndrome.

3. In spite of her very marked deficits in speeded eye–hand coordination on novel tasks, Cathy's cursive script was excellent, as can be seen in the spelling sample in Figure 7.2. This would certainly attest to the crystallized nature of this skill, which was, at this point in her development, probably being mediated by systems within the left cerebral hemisphere. In this sample of her handwriting from the WRAT Spelling

subtest, note might be taken of the extremely high level of phonetic accuracy of her misspellings and her frequent failure to cross t's, and dot i's. The degree of neglect of the left side of visual space suggested by the latter is seen frequently in persons with brain lesions similar to those sustained by Cathy.

4. It is clear that Cathy experienced very marked difficulties in nonverbal concept formation, strategy generation, and hypothesis testing, as exemplified by her markedly impaired level of performance on the Category Test. It is notable that she had considerable difficulty with all aspects of this test, including the last subtest, which is made up of items from the previous subtests. Her problems in benefiting from informational feedback were especially evident on this test. Another example of her difficulties in nonverbal problem solving can be seen on the Tactual Performance Test, especially her apparent failure to benefit from experience with this task. In the first examination, she took 10.41 minutes to place all six blocks with her right hand on the first trial, and 9.78 minutes to place the six blocks with both (primarily right) hands on a third trial. This failure to exhibit a positive transfer-of-training effect on complex nonverbal problem-solving tasks is quite typical of youngsters with NLD.

5. A comparison of her normal scores on the Speech-Sounds Perception Test (first examination) and the WISC Digit Span subtest (both examinations), with her markedly impaired score on the Target Test (both examinations) would certainly suggest that her capacities for auditory attention and immediate memory were much better than were her capacities for visual attention and immediate memory. In the first examination, her normal level of incidental memory for the blocks used on the Tactual Performance Test was probably a function of her capacity to name the blocks; this would, undoubtedly, aid her memory for them. In the same examination, her markedly impaired capacity to locate her drawings of the blocks in their proper locations on a drawing of the formboard used for the Tactual Performance Test may be a function of her problems in dealing with visual-spatial relationships and/or difficulties in visual imagery. Such problems continued in the second examination; however, her considerably lower level of tolerance for frustration at the time of the second examination rendered the interpretation of her performance at that time somewhat problematic.

6. Performance on the WISC Similarities and Digit Span subtests was within normal limits. Normal performance was also in evidence on the Speech-Sounds Perception Test (first examination) and the Auditory Closure Test (second examination). Levels of performance on the Sen-

tence Memory and Verbal Fluency Tests were clearly impaired in both examinations. This pattern of differences is expected to obtain in the NLD syndrome; that is, we expect relatively normal performance on rote and verbal tasks and relatively impaired performance on tasks (even verbal ones) that place a premium on understanding (e.g., memory for meaningful sentences) and those that are somewhat novel (e.g., phonemically cued verbal fluency). In a word, her performance on the Sentence Memory Test would appear to suggest an inability to utilize contextual cues as an aid in the recall of nonredundant verbal information; her immediate and/or short-term recall for rote material (e.g., digits) was not affected by her impairment in the higher-order, pragmatic aspects of language.

7. The following examples of stability and change are of interest. Mild oral-motor praxis difficulties were evident in both examinations. There was a significant increase in PPVT performance between the two testings. (With respect to her very low levels of performance on the PPVT in both testings, it should be pointed out that the PPVT, although designed as a test of receptive vocabulary, involves accurate visual scanning of four visual alternatives before deciding upon a correct response for the orally delivered target word. This type of visual search, especially within the left visual field, was not an activity at which Cathy was very adept. Indeed, for her, the PPVT turned out to be more of a reflection of her deficiencies in visual scanning and related skills than of her receptive vocabulary.) Her misspellings were almost exclusively of the phonetically accurate variety in both testings. These particular examples of stability and change are quite typical of those seen in the NLD syndrome. In this particular case, we see an example of a youngster whose adaptive abilities and deficits are moving toward the more typical manifestations of the NLD syndrome as the acute effects of her brain lesions subside.

8. Cathy's particular *pattern* of high WRAT Reading and Spelling and low Arithmetic is a hallmark of the older child or the adolescent who exhibits NLD. Note that, within fairly broad limits, it is the *pattern* rather than the *levels* of performance that are crucial in this regard. As we saw in the case of Mary, and will see again in the case of John, it matters little or not at all whether any of the scores on these three subtests are within, below, or above the normal range; the crucial interpretive dimension is the *difference* between reading and spelling on the one hand and arithmetic on the other.

9. At the time of the first examination, Cathy's general level of affect was quite flat and expressionless. This was also evident in the second

examination. In addition, it was abundantly clear by the time of the second examination that she was developing a rather serious level of socioemotional disturbance. Previously very popular with her agemates, she was, by the time of the second testing, all but shunned by them. Part of this was a function of the fact that most of her previous friends had gone on to Secondary School, whereas she had been left behind in Elementary School. However, there was an added set of problems occasioned by her frequent displays of inappropriate behavior, her essentially repetitive and virtually content-free utterances, and her failure to communicate affectively or to appreciate such communications from others. The latter difficulties rendered association with her a rather unreinforcing condition for virtually all of her former friends and associates. This set of difficulties—being "held back" in school and exhibiting the type of interpersonal behavior that we have come to associate with NLD youngsters—is quite typical of severely head-injured children and adolescents.

The most prominent feature of Cathy's adaptive ability structure was her rather pronounced impairment on those tests that require perception, memory, analysis, synthesis, and integration of visual-spatial information. In addition, it was clear that her capacity to engage in tasks that involved relatively novel, complex concept-formation and problem-solving abilities was also significantly impaired. The relatively slight improvement in her performance in these areas over the two test sessions may have reflected (1) some adaptation to the left-visual-field neglect that was in evidence during both examinations and (2) some improvement in general visual attention skills. As we might expect in an individual who has experienced a rather significant amount of tissue loss from the right temporal and adjacent parietal regions, this girl continued to exhibit impaired sensory functioning on the left side of her body. However, it should be noted that there was some improvement in her psychomotor skills, especially with the left hand, and we would normally expect that such skills would continue to improve to some extent, especially with treatment. (Recall that the right frontal lobe was essentially spared in this case.)

Note on Neuropsychological Interpretation. It should be borne in mind that one cannot rule out the possibility of left-hemisphere involvement in this case, particularly in view of the severe head trauma that this girl experienced. Contre-coup effects, for example, are quite common in cases such as this. In addition, the swelling noted during surgery, which necessitated excision of large portions of the right cerebral hemisphere, could easily have resulted in damage to more remote areas of the cortex. The improvements noted in some aspects of motor skills with the right hand and in verbal fluency over the 6-month period between the two testings may reflect some recovery of function of the anterior regions of the left cerebral hemisphere. At the same time, there are good reasons to believe that Cathy will continue to experience considerable difficulty on novel word-finding tasks, for reasons that are essentially distinct from the degree of dysfunction in the anterior regions of the left cerebral hemisphere.

MARY AND CATHY: SOME COMPARISONS

By now, I am sure that the reader has noted a number of similarities and differences between the neuropsychological presentations of Mary and Cathy. One particularly interesting difference is that evident in their graphomotor performances (see Figures 7.1 and 7.2). Note that Mary's printing is large, tremulous, and quite uncoordinated, whereas Cathy's is of normal size, steady, and flowing. This difference might be interpreted as reflecting the essentially normal period of development that Cathy experienced prior to her brain insult, as compared to the "developmental" difficulties faced by Mary in all areas of eye–hand coordination. Note that both youngsters exhibited markedly impaired performances on novel psychomotor tasks (e.g., Grooved Pegboard Test); this attests to the fact that both, at the time of testing, had difficulties in such situations. The interesting aspect of Cathy's performance is the virtually complete preservation of coordinated cursive script, in spite of the latter limitations.

Theoretically, the importance of this dissociation is the likely reasons for it. In terms of the NLD model, it would be inferred that, for Cathy, cursive script had become automatized well before the onset of her brain lesion. This automatization, in turn, would be expected to imply that left-hemisphere systems had "taken over" the writing function prior to the brain lesion. Since the lesion was confined to the right cerebral hemisphere (and, possibly, some aspects of the anterior regions of the left hemisphere), this would imply that systems in these brain regions can be dysfunctional while cursive script, if previously automatized, remains intact. The fact that other skills thought to be subserved primarily by systems within the temporo-parietal region of the left cerebral hemisphere (e.g., speech-sounds perception) were also at normal or above-normal levels at the time of the first examination would raise the possibility that these same systems may be primarily responsible for mediating cursive script at this stage in Cathy's development.

With respect to an evaluation of the similarities in the neuropsychological profiles of Mary and Cathy, one need only examine the assets and deficits expected to be present in the NLD syndrome. This would lead to a determination that these two youngsters were, indeed, remarkably similar in their neuropsychological presentations. The following case also illustrates the rather homogeneous neuropsychological presentations of such youngsters, this time in a youngster who did not present with any clearly demonstrable brain disease.

CASE 3: JANE[4]

The two previous cases illustrated the features of the NLD syndrome in youngsters with well-documented brain disease. In the case of Jane, we have an example of a "developmental" presentation of the NLD syndrome. As is outlined in the following discussion, she did not exhibit any "hard" signs of neurological disease; however, there were deviations (mostly slowness) in development that occasioned concern over her neurological well-being.

Jane underwent comprehensive neuropsychological evaluations on four occasions: at the ages of 9 years, 6 months; 11 years, 0 months; 12 years, 11 months; and 15 years, 5 months. She was also examined on a more circumscribed basis at the age of 17 years, 8 months. The presentation of findings in this case concentrates on the first and fourth comprehensive neuropsychological assessments. A brief review of the evaluation at 11 years, 0 months is also included. Only the VABS results at 17 years, 8 months are reported formally. Of particular importance in this presentation is the stability of Jane's neuropsychological status over time, the evidence of her positive response to a program of therapy/intervention, and her residual difficulties in adaptive functioning at the age of almost 18 years.

---

[4]Aspects of this case have been presented previously, in Rourke, Bakker, et al. (1983), pp. 238–247.

Relevant History

This youngster was referred for neuropsychological assessment by her family physician. She was said to be experiencing problems in communicating through writing, and her mechanical arithmetic skills were reported to be very weak. In addition, it was reported that her fine and gross motor abilities were very poorly developed. On the other hand, her oral reading and spelling abilities were described as quite good. At the time of the initial assessment, she was 9½ years of age and was enrolled in a regular Grade 4 program. Her mother reported that Jane had difficulties with concentration, and she also expressed concern regarding her ability to relate to other children.

Inspection of Jane's history revealed that she was the firstborn child, delivered by caesarian section after a full-term pregnancy and an unsuccessful trial of labor. The child was nursed for 24 hours in an incubator and later on in a normal crib. For the most part, Jane's infancy was unremarkable, although at 14 months of age it was noted that her motor coordination and vocabulary were somewhat delayed. She had no serious illnesses during infancy and childhood, except for a few febrile episodes, during one or two of which she became somewhat delirious. She was also under medical care for possible allergies.

Behavioral Observations during the Examinations

During the initial daylong assessment (at 9 years, 6 months), Jane was reasonably cooperative and friendly with the examiner; rapport was easily established with her. However, she seemed to be somewhat distractible, exhibiting difficulties with attentional deployment. She often required guidance and encouragement in order to exert her best efforts; the exception to this was her rather enthusiastic approach to tasks of a clearly verbal, especially academic, nature. She required considerable instruction, assistance, and practice in order to complete motoric and visual-spatial tasks as required. She was quite loquacious; however, her conversation was rather inappropriate, tangential, and often unrelated to the task at hand. Her gait was awkward, and her general level of motor coordination was noticeably poor. It should be clear from this description of her ambient behavior during this examination that she exhibited many characteristics that we have come to associate with children who exhibit the NLD syndrome.

Throughout the second examination at the age of 11 years, 0 months (which is not reported in full here), she was reasonably friendly, talkative, and cooperative; rapport was easily obtained with her. However, there was some evidence of slight distractibility and carelessness, and on some occasions she seemed to give up on tasks that she perceived as too difficult. It was fairly obvious from her performance on paper-and-pencil tasks that her eye–hand coordination was quite poor. She seemed to have particular difficulty in starting lines on the left side of the page, apparently because she experienced problems in controlling her hand movement from the end of one line (on the right side) to the beginning of the next line (on the left side). Another notable feature of her behavior in this second examination was a rather different, "sing-song" quality to her voice.

In the fourth examination at the age of 15 years, 5 months, Jane was very cooperative and very talkative. Her motivation to do well on the tests administered was never in any doubt. In general, she was somewhat hypoactive. Occasionally, she became a bit distracted from the task at hand; this took the form of "drifting off" during passive attending conditions, when she seemed to be unaware that stimuli were being presented to her. It is notable that this distractibility was confined almost exclusively to those situations involving the presentation of visual stimuli. Her general level of motor coordination, especially when walking or engaged in fine manipulatory activities, was quite awkward. On several occasions she exhibited rather immature behavior, although her general approach to the testing situation was one of compliance and cooperation. Again, her ambient behavior at the time of this fourth testing was quite typical of that seen in NLD adolescents.

Neurological Examination Results at 10 Years

The electroencephalographic (EEG) evaluation Jane underwent at age 10 was not particularly helpful. The tracing obtained was judged to be essentially within normal limits, except for some nonspecific, generalized mild dysrhythmia emanating from both cerebral hemispheres. Activation did not provoke any focal abnormality or epileptic activity. Physical neurological examination revealed mild ataxia and apraxia, with the latter appearing to be more marked on the left side. She also exhibited a marked nystagmus on gaze to the left. Otherwise, the neurological examination was unremarkable. On the basis of these findings, the neurologist suggested possible mild cerebellar–pontine dysfunction. A question was also raised regarding possible endocrine dysfunction, because of the generalized distribution of adipose tissue.

Treatment/Intervention Program

Following her first neuropsychological assessment, Jane entered a day-treatment program on a full-time basis. She spent 5 years in this program. Following this experience, she was enrolled in a residential treatment program for approximately 2 years. In both programs there was a heavy emphasis on life-skills training, psychomotor development, counseling, and appropriate-level academic training. Especially during the initial 5-year day-treatment placement, these efforts were guided by the principles and procedures outlined in the general treatment/intervention program that is presented toward the end of this chapter. It is important to emphasize the intensive nature of the treatment programs in which Jane was involved over the 7-year period in question, when interpreting the neuropsychological assessment results available during this time frame.

Discussion: NLD Elements and Dynamics

The results of Jane's first and fourth neuropsychological assessments are summarized in Figure 7.3. In the first of these, at 9 years, 6 months of age, it was quite clear that Jane exhibited the major neuropsychological, academic, and socioemotional features of the NLD syndrome. Indeed, there were few deviations from this pattern in evidence. In view of this, the treatment/intervention program just discussed was commenced; it was implemented while Jane was enrolled in day-treatment in a center specializing in the care of learning-disabled children who have associated mental health needs.

The results of the second examination, at 11 years, 0 months (not included in the figure), indicated that she had made considerable gains in a number of areas of adaptive functioning. The most notable of these were in the areas of motor steadiness, motor coordination, problem-solving attack strategies, spelling, and some elements of attentional deployment. It was equally clear, however, that she continued to experience rather marked visual-spatial-organizational difficulties, together with

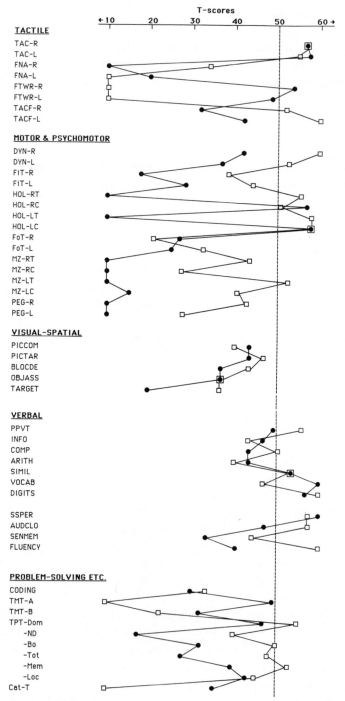

FIGURE 7.3. Summary of Jane's neuropsychological test results. ●—●, first testing; □—□, fourth testing.

	Testing 1 (9 yr, 6 mo)	Testing 4 (15 yr, 5 mo)
WISC		
VIQ	101	101
PIQ	75	79
FSIQ	88	90
Underlining (no. of each)		
Superior	n.a.	2
Average	n.a.	5
Borderline	n.a.	1
Mild	n.a.	4
Moderate	n.a.	1
Severe	n.a.	0
Speed subtest	n.a.	Mild
WRAT (grade; centile)		
Reading	9.3; 99.3	9.9; 84
Spelling	6.5; 86	9.5; 73
Arithmetic	3; 16	4.6; 7
PIC (*T* score)		
Lie	53	45
F	80	63
Defensiveness	29	43
Adjustment	75	81
Achievement	62	69
Intellectual Screening	100	100
Development	79	73
Somatic Concern	73	66
Depression	62	71
Family Relations	47	41
Delinquency	51	69
Withdrawal	58	73
Anxiety	60	55
Psychosis	105	78
Hyperactivity	53	49
Social Skills	66	73
ARS		
No	13	20
Little	12	7
Very much	7	0
BPC		
No	29	30
Little	28	35
Very much	8	1

FIGURE 7.3. (continued)

APHASIA SCREENING TEST
In the first examination, Jane exhibited difficulties in simple arithmetic calculation; however, there were no errors in simple arithmetic exhibited at 15 years, 5 months. In both examinations, Jane exhibited mild difficulty in the enunciation of complex, multisyllabic words. Otherwise, her performance on this test was unremarkable.

EXAMPLE FROM WRAT SPELLING SUBTEST

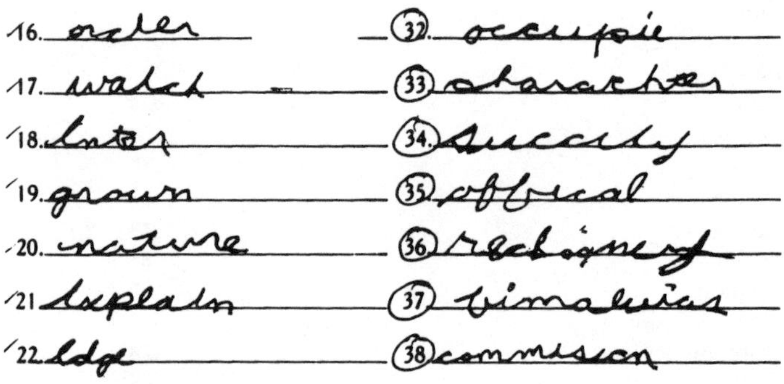

problems in short-term memory for visual sequences. Although her drawings of geometric forms remained slightly distorted, there were indications of some improvement in her capacity to organize visual-spatial output. While eye–hand coordination improved somewhat, it remained enough of a problem for her that her performance under speeded conditions continued to be an area of concern. As was observed in the first assessment, Jane exhibited rather well-developed skills in reading (word recognition) and spelling, but arithmetic remained an area of relative academic weakness. She was able to add, subtract, and multiply in a competent manner, but division still posed difficulty for her.

As a result of this second assessment, it was felt that a continuation of her therapeutic program was in order. There was every indication that the specific training that commenced at the conclusion of the first assessment seemed to have helped her in many areas of adaptive functioning; at the very least, there were no compelling indications of deterioration in her most deficient areas of adaptive functioning.

Aside from her obvious academic difficulties, especially in the area of arithmetic, a major problem faced by Jane involved her poorly developed social skills. Indeed, at the age of 12 years, she obtained a social age equivalent to 8.3 years and a social quotient of 69 on the Vineland Social Maturity Scale (Doll, 1953). Personnel at the treatment center in which she was enrolled described her as being friendly with adults and tending to seek their praise and acknowledgment in an active manner. They also reported, however, that she responded to social interactions in a rather automatic fashion, with only a limited expression of meaningful affect. Her relationships with peers were certainly less than ideal, often characterized by silly, inappropriate talk on her part.

It is clear that the major factor in Jane's poorly developed social skills related to her inability to interpret appropriate nonverbal sources of communication, such as facial expressions, body postures, and various gestures. She would be expected to be at considerable risk for misinterpreting or failing to interpret many relevant elements in social situations.

Despite the difficulties that Jane exhibited at 11 and 12 years of age, it was also clear that the intensive treatment program provided for her had paid some dividends. Test–retest comparisons indicated dramatic improvements in her motor and psychomotor skills. In addition, it was quite clear that her capacity to attend to auditory stimulation had increased, although this did not appear to be the case within the visual-spatial or tactile-perceptual realm. Visual scanning and tracking remained a problem, and, while this did not appear to affect the reading of single words, it may have interfered with her capacity to extract meaning from reading passages. It was evident that Jane was very adept at associating and defining words, although the associations that she made to words often tended to be rather bizarre.

Prior to treatment, she had very few positive socializing experiences outside of her immediate family. Her experience in the treatment program, in addition to providing an opportunity to develop her academic skills, undoubtedly contributed to a better social experience for her. Because of the many gains that Jane exhibited as a result of treatment, plans were formulated to find a placement for her in a regular school system. Unfortunately, this did not turn out to be a clinically viable tack to follow. Indeed, reports from her parents and her caretakers in the treatment program continued to indicate that she was not "ready" to take this step. Trials of partial integration within the regular school system were orchestrated carefully and with considerable cooperation from the school in question; however, repeated observations by all of those involved in her care led to the conclusion that Jane would need the support of a treatment center and program for the foreseeable future.

In order to cast some light on why this turned out to be the case, it would be instructive to consider the results of Jane's fourth neuropsychological assessment, at 15 year, 5 months (see Figure 7.3). These are best described in terms of a set of comparisons with the results obtained in her first assessment, as follows:

1. In general, the results of the first and fourth examinations were quite similar. This was especially apparent in the areas of Jane's principal neuropsychological deficiencies, as measured with the Performance subtests of the WISC and with the Category Test (the adult version was administered in the fourth examination).

2. It should be noted that there were some changes in a positive direction in some of her expected areas of neuropsychological strength, such as simple motor skills (e.g., grip strength; finger tapping speed), rote verbal skills (e.g., WISC Digit Span, Auditory Closure Test), and other verbal receptive skills (e.g., PPVT).

3. The areas where it is thought that her therapy/intervention program may have been most helpful included her improved performance on the Tactual Performance Test. However, note should be taken of the persistence since the first assessment of the pattern of relative performance deficiency with the left hand.

4. The persistence of Jane's patterns of performance over time is quite remarkable, especially when one considers that this occurred in the academic areas (high reading and spelling versus low arithmetic), the "verbal" versus visual-spatial-organizational areas, and patterns of socioemotional responsivity.

5. With respect to the latter, however, it should be noted that Jane's PIC results do reflect some encouraging gains. See especially the much lower elevation on the Psychosis scale and the general ebbing of those factors that contribute to the PIC internalized psychopathology factor.

Jane's clinical picture at the time of her fourth assessment contained a number of rather significant and encouraging positive developments that, presumably, were a function of the rather intensive therapy/intervention program in which she had been participating. However, the VABS results at the time of her fifth testing (see Figure 7.4) were not reflective of a capacity for completely independent living at that time. These results are, indeed, somewhat discouraging, in that they point to a number of adaptive areas within which Jane had made precious little progress over time. More generally, it is often the case that the VABS

FIGURE 7.4. Jane's Vineland Adaptive Behavior Scale scores at 17 years, 8 months (fifth assessment).

	Standard score	Centile	Age-equivalent score
Communication	48	<1	8 yr, 10 mo
Daily Living	57	<1	8 yr, 10 mo
Socialization	47	<1	5 yr, 11 mo
Motor (estimates)			4 yr, 3 mo
Adaptive Behavior Composite	47	<1	
Maladaptive Scale (raw score: 22; significant)			

FIGURE 7.5. Gerry's Vineland Adaptive Behavior Scale scores at 16 years, 4 months.

	Standard score	Centile	Age-equivalent score
Communication	70	2	10 yr, 10 mo
Daily Living	78	7	11 yr, 9 mo
Socialization	69	2	10 yr, 4 mo
Motor (estimates)	103	58	>5 yr, 11 mo
Adaptive Behavior Composite	67	1	11 yr, 0 mo
Maladaptive Scale (raw score: 13; significant)			

results of NLD youngsters are more pervasively and more significantly impaired than are those of their brain-damaged agemates who have sustained very significant cerebral lesions that have not had a widespread negative impact on white matter functioning.

Jane and Gerry: Social/Vocational Outcomes

In order to illustrate the latter point, the VABS results of a 16-year-old youngster, Gerry, are reported in Figure 7.5. This boy had sustained a very severe stroke involving the middle region of the left cerebral hemisphere. The bleeding and subsequent necrosis of tissue within this region left him with very severe aphasiological symptomatology (similar to the disconnection syndrome) and marked motoric limitations on the right side of the body. In spite of these deficiencies, we note that his VABS scores are generally superior to Jane's. (For a more complete analysis of this particular case, see Chapter 2 of Rourke, Fisk, & Strang, 1986.)

In light of these differences, it is instructive to consider and compare Jane's and Gerry's current social and vocational status. At the age of 20, Jane is involved in a "career search" that is proceeding reasonably well. She is receiving considerable support in this effort from a number of individuals, including her parents. She is thought to have achieved a marginal level of adjustment, but the earmarks of the NLD syndrome, especially in the areas of judgment and reasoning, persist. It is clear that her deficiencies in these areas will continue to impose substantial limitations on her social and vocational life. Gerry, at the age of 20, is still quite frankly aphasic; however, he is seen as quite well adjusted and socially adaptive. One pursuit in which he has been engaged has involved assisting handicapped individuals in the use of computers as part of their therapy programs. Gerry is quite adept at this teaching enterprise and is well liked by his students. His own computer is programed with a variety of software that he can access on demand when his word-finding skills fail him. He is quite adept at deciding when he needs access to such material and manages to do so without alienating those around him. These few observations should be sufficient to suggest that the modes of adaptation for Jane and Gerry are quite different, and that the prognosis for social and vocational adjustment is significantly more positive for Gerry than for Jane.

JANE, MARY, AND CATHY: SOME COMPARISONS

In comparing Jane's neuropsychological protocol with those of Mary and Cathy, it is clear that there are a number of similarities in the patterns of test results obtained. In all three cases, the children presented with impaired visual-spatial skills, some tactile-perceptual difficulties, deficient problem-solving and concept-formation abilities, impaired psychomotor functioning, and relatively intact rote verbal skills. Cathy, however, exhibited clearly lateralized sensory-perceptual and motor signs, and her level of psychometric intelligence was inconsistent with the level of academic performance obtained on the WRAT. In these and other ways, her protocol was entirely in keeping with the acute phase of the brain lesions that she had sustained. Her clinical history, in addition to the medical data, supported the view that the presenting problem was a result of relatively recent neurological trauma. For Jane, the motor and sensory impairments observed were more bilateral and less lateralized and somewhat less severe than those exhibited by Cathy. With respect to severity, Jane did not exhibit any simple tactile or auditory imperception and there was no clear evidence of visual-field defects. However, she frequently made more errors on the left than on the right side of the page when doing tasks such as the Underlining Test. In comparison to Mary, Jane's neuropsychological test results were also of a somewhat less severe nature; however, the pattern of scores exhibited by these two youngsters is remarkably similar.

The principal point to be made in this connection is that Jane's *pattern* of test results is quite typical of the "developmental" presentation of the NLD syndrome. However, in spite of her somewhat better *levels* of performance, she is still facing social and vocational difficulties that we would fully expect Mary and Cathy to encounter. Although it would appear to be the case that Jane's therapy/intervention program has been quite successful in a number of areas, it is clear that she still experiences very significant limitations in her adaptive capacities, as an apparent reflection of the NLD syndrome.

CASE 4: JOHN

John's neuropsychological, academic, and social features also reflect the developmental presentation of the NLD syndrome. Our consideration of his neuropsychological status will focus on the results of his second assessment at the age of 12 years, 11 months; the results of his first assessment at the age of 11 are presented for comparison purposes only.

The reasons for the importance of this case relate to the misunderstandings that can frequently obtain on the part of otherwise quite prudent and thoughtful caretakers of the NLD child. The dimensions of repression and denial on the part of parents and other caretakers regarding the actual assets and deficits of such youngsters occur often enough to be thought typical. The dynamics of John's neuropsychological presentation, in concert with his academic and social performance, illustrate the potential for such sources of counterproductive mismanagement.

Note on Presentation. John's results are couched in a fashion very similar to that used in the typical report presentation that we employ for such youngsters. It is hoped that this mode of presentation will be of some assistance to the reader who is interested in neuropsychological reporting style.

Background

This boy of almost 13 years was referred for his second neuropsychological assessment in order to determine the nature and extent of his adaptive skills and abilities. He was reported to have difficulties in academic subjects in the sciences and in social relationships outside the home. At the time of this assessment, his parents were particularly interested in determining which therapeutic modalities would be preferrable for their son, and whether he needed some form of alternative education.

Behavioral Observations during the Examination

Although this boy was generally cooperative with the examiner, rapport was very difficult to obtain and maintain with him. He was very taciturn throughout the examination, and he made eye contact with the examiner only when absolutely necessary. He exhibited an average response speed and an average level of general physical activity. For the most part, he resisted guessing in situations where he was unsure of an answer. His general demeanor was shy and withdrawn, and it was difficult to ascertain his precise level of motivation for many of the tests administered to him.

On many tasks requiring visual search, he tended to work very close to the stimulus materials. On one test for ocular dominance, it was noted that he squinted at the stimulus materials and misnamed 3 of the 10 simple objects. It appeared from this performance that his visual status needed to be evaluated and monitored. It was reported later, however, that his corrective lenses, which he was wearing during the examination, were sufficient to compensate for his ocular acuity difficulties.

Throughout the examination, this boy made no more eye contact with the examiner than was absolutely necessary. His facial expression was flat and uncommunicative. There were many occasions when he became quite fidgety. The one repetitive behavior in which he was noted to engage was constantly examining the face of his wristwatch, which was set at 4 hours behind the actual time of day.

All things considered, it would appear probable that we obtained a fairly reliable estimate of this boy's adaptive skills and abilities in this examination.

Summary of Test Results and Impressions

John's test results are summarized in Figure 7.6. As can be seen, this boy exhibited a very evident pattern of impaired visual-spatial-organizational skills, eye–hand coordination difficulties, tactile-perceptual deficits, and higher-level nonverbal concept-formation difficulties, within a context of some well-developed, automatic, rote verbal skills. Children who exhibit this pattern of abilities and deficits are almost always very much at risk for the development of serious degrees of internalized psychopathology, usually marked by depression, withdrawal, high levels of anxiety, and extreme difficulties in social skills. With the possible exception of ostensible anxiety, this boy would appear to be suffering from these expected effects. Also, such children typically have much more difficulty with mechanical arithmetic than with word recognition and spelling; and considerable difficulties with concept formation, problem solving, and scientific thinking. All of these features appear to characterize John's behavior. The following sections of this report were designed to add some specifications to these generalizations and to offer some suggestions for intervention for him in the academic and therapeutic milieux.

There were no indications of any tactile imperception or suppression. There was clear evidence of finger agnosia and finger dysgraphesthesia with the right hand. John exhibited very evident astereognosis for coins bilaterally; however, he had no difficulty in recognizing the visual representations of simpler forms by touch.

On a complex nonverbal problem-solving task (TPT) involving psychomotor coordination, strategy generation, and the capacity to benefit from tactile input and kinesthetic feedback, his overall level of performance was markedly impaired. Although he appeared to benefit in a limited way from continued experience with this task, his performance on the second and third trials, using his left hand for the former and both hands, for the latter, were particularly poor. His incidental memory for the shapes and locations of the blocks used on this task was extremely poor.

There were no indications of any auditory imperception or suppression. Performance on a Sweep Hearing Test was negative. He performed within normal limits on a task requiring fine auditory discrimination and sustained attention (Seashore Rhythm Test).

His levels of performance were superior on tests for speech-sounds perception, sound blending, and sentence memory. However, his level of performance on a phonemically cued test of verbal fluency was mildly

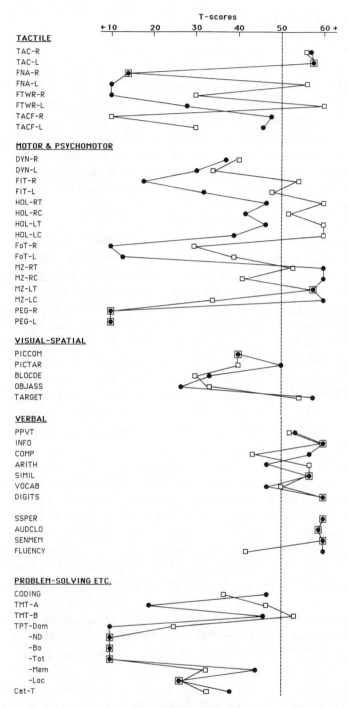

FIGURE 7.6. Summary of John's neuropsychological test results. ●—●, first testing; □—□, second testing.

	Testing 1 (11 yr, 0 mo)	Testing 2 (12 yr, 11 mo)
WISC		
VIQ	107	106
PIQ	78	72
FSIQ	92	88
Underlining (no. of each)		
Superior	1	1
Average	3	3
Borderline	1	1
Mild	2	5
Moderate	5	1
Severe	1	2
Speed subtest	Moderate	Borderline
WRAT (grade; centile)		
Reading	8+; 95	12+; 99
Spelling	8+; 98	12+; 95
Arithmetic	4; 21	9; 68
PIC (T score)		
Lie	45	42
F	69	71
Defensiveness	41	37
Adjustment	65	79
Achievement	57	74
Intellectual Screening	72	100
Development	65	82
Somatic Concern	67	42
Depression	81	51
Family Relations	47	43
Delinquency	59	55
Withdrawal	76	65
Anxiety	79	48
Psychosis	112	92
Hyperactivity	31	39
Social Skills	67	77
ARS		
No	n.a.	19
Little	n.a.	5
Very much	n.a.	8
BPC		
No	n.a.	49
Little	n.a.	11
Very much	n.a.	6

	Standard score	Centile	Age-equivalent score
VABS (at 11½ yr only)			
Communication	61	<1	7 yr, 2 mo
Daily Living	27	<1	4 yr, 6 mo
Socialization	54	<1	4 yr, 6 mo
Motor		<1	3 yr, 7 mo
Adaptive Behavior Composite	44	<1	4 yr, 11 mo

FIGURE 7.6. (continued)

APHASIA SCREENING TEST
There were no frankly aphasic signs in evidence in either examination; however, John expressed confusion in both administrations of this test when asked to place his left hand to his left elbow. He did not appear to understand that this was impossible and continued to try to think of a way to accomplish this feat.

EXAMPLE FROM WRAT SPELLING SUBTEST

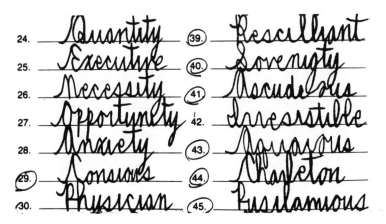

impaired. It would appear probable that the rather novel nature of the latter task was the feature of it that posed particular difficulty for him.

There was no clear evidence of any aphasic deficits on the Aphasia Screening Test; however, John did express considerable confusion when an obviously nonsensical direction regarding orientation and understanding of his own body was delivered. It was also noted that, in writing the word *warning*, he did not place a dot over the i in it.

On the WISC-R he obtained a Verbal IQ of 106. Subtest scaled scores on this section ranged from a low of 8 on the Comprehension subtest to a high of 19 on the Digit Span subtest. Thus it is evident that John found it much easier to deal with rote material that he needed only to repeat or recall in a verbatim fashion than he did to deal with the understanding of the implications of verbal discourse. This would appear to be a fairly general characteristic of his behavior in situations calling for verbal understanding and responding.

On the Peabody Picture Vocabulary Test he obtained a Mental Age of 13 years, 11 months, which is equivalent to an IQ of 103. It is notable that this test, designed as a measure of single-word receptive vocabulary, yields a result virtually identical to that evident on the Verbal section of the WISC-R.

There were no indications of any visual imperception or suppression. John performed within normal limits on a task requiring immediate memory for visual sequences (Target Test).

His graphic renderings of simple visual designs were marked by mild visual-spatial distortions and a mild degree of tremor. His graphic rendering of a complex key was quite oversimplified and immature. It was the sort of drawing that is often made by children who experience considerable difficulty in appreciating fine visual detail. His cursive script was somewhat large, but the letters were reasonably well formed. It is notable that he almost never placed dots on the letter "i," but that he did cross the letter "t" when writing. The finer visual detail of the former may be crucial in this respect.

This boy did not experience any particular difficulty on a task that required him to search through a series of numbered and lettered circles, join them together in order, and switch back and forth between the numeric and alphabetic sequences in so doing. This and other observations in the current examination would suggest that he had some potential for directing his behavior in terms of memorized verbal rules and procedures.

On the Underlining Test, John had particular difficulty with those subtests that involved complex visual stimuli as target and distractor items. He did much better on those items involving verbal targets and distractors, although sequencing problems were evident in some of these instances.

On the WISC-R he obtained a Performance IQ of 72. Subtest scaled scores on this section ranged from a low of 4 on the Block Design subtest and 5 on the Object Assembly subtest to highs of 7 on the Picture Completion and Picture Arrangement subtests. It is evident that he had considerable difficulty with visual-spatial analysis, organization, and synthesis, especially in situations where speeded responses were required.

This boy would appear to be exclusively right-handed, right-footed, and right-eyed. Strength of grip was roughly normal with the upper extremities. The same situation obtained with respect to motor speed with each hand. Motor speed with the feet was somewhat slowed bilaterally. John did not experience any difficulties on a task specifically designed for the measurement of static steadiness; however, he did experience some mild difficulties on a test for kinetic steadiness. His levels of performance were markedly impaired on a test requiring fine motor coordination under speeded conditions (Grooved Pegboard Test); performance with the left hand on this test was particularly impaired. Thus, this boy experienced increasing difficulty in the motoric sphere as the requirements for eye–hand coordination increased. This difficulty became exacerbated dramatically under speeded conditions and/or in situations that required the integration of information from more than one sensory modality.

On a very complex nonverbal concept-formation task (Category Test) involving hypothesis testing, strategy generation, problem solving, and the capacity to benefit from positive and negative informational feedback) this boy's overall level of performance was moderately impaired. His incidental memory for previously correct solutions on this task was also moderately impaired.

On the WRAT-R he obtained the following approximate grade-equivalent and centile scores, respectively: Reading (word-recognition), 12(99); Spelling, 12(95); and Arithmetic, 9(68). On the Spelling test virtually all of his misspellings were of the phonetically accurate variety, as would be expected in view of his performance on tests for speech-sounds perception and auditory blending, mentioned earlier. He also showed himself well able to utilize a phonetic word-attack strategy for the decoding of novel words. Most of his arithmetic calculations were carried out quite systematically; however, there was some inattention to visual detail evident in some of these calculations.

Summary and Recommendations

Although clearly not diagnostic of any neuropathological condition, this particular profile of neuropsychological results is often seen in children of this age who are suffering from significant impairment in skills and abilities ordinarily thought to be subserved primarily by systems within the right cerebral hemisphere. In addition, subcortical and diffuse white matter dysfunction is often found to be implicated in such cases. This profile would not be consistent with the presence of an acute neurological disease; rather, this pattern of skills, abilities, and deficiencies is most often seen in children suffering from a chronic, developmental disability.

The ramifications of this particular pattern of abilities and deficits are far-reaching, usually affecting every aspect of academic and social life. Hence, the therapeutic programs necessary to handle these difficulties are always quite complex and need to be quite comprehensive and integrated. In this connection, I should point out that the Personality Inventory for Children completed by John's father yielded a profile that is typical of this syndrome, namely, much internalized psychopathology, problems noted throughout the developmental course, and difficulties in social judgment and social learning. Treatment within a center for the emotionally disturbed is often recommended for children such as this, but one has to be very cautious with such a recommendation because it is usually the case that the therapeutic personnel within such a center are naive with respect to the social, emotional, and academic implications of the NLD syndrome.

General Conclusions and Recommendations Regarding Intervention

Specific avenues to pursue in the therapeutic management of this child (modeled after the program outlined toward the end of this chapter) were discussed in detail at a conference convened soon after the neuropsychological assessment under consideration. The parents seemed receptive to the therapeutic program proposed and to the alterations in the educational program that were recommended. However, it was learned soon after this conference that the principal mode of intervention that was secured for this boy was one that could best be described as psychodynamic in orientation, with much emphasis being given to insight-oriented psychotherapeutic treatment.

As pointed out in previous sections of this work, such forms of therapy tend to be quite counterproductive for persons who exhibit the NLD syndrome. They are usually opted for because even reasonably astute observers tend to overvalue the "intelligence" of NLD adolescents. This is also the principal reason for an unwillingness to adopt an approach to formal educational intervention that would increase the NLD youngster's probability of success. Such an approach usually involves dimensions such as avoiding the teaching of science in the usual manner and encouraging compensations that would accentuate areas of rote memory assets and minimize the necessity for deploying the NLD youngster's impaired concept-formation, judgment, and reasoning abilities.

It should be emphasized that it is quite easy for caretakers of NLD children and adolescents to overestimate grossly their capacities for adaptation and learning of virtually every sort. Apparently well-developed verbal abilities, very infrequently examined from the point of view of their content and pragmatics, often lead such caretakers to the view that, once underlying psychic conflicts have been resolved, the energy needed to be outstandingly successful in school and elsewhere will be available and applied by the NLD child or adolescent. Unfortunately, this never turns out to be the case.

CASE 5: BOB

There are three features of this case presentation that should be emphasized: It involves the examination of a child much younger than those discussed previously; the child was suffering from the effects of a severe craniocerebral trauma sustained during an early developmental stage; and there was some litigation surrounding this case. Furthermore, so as to reflect rather directly the clinical realities of actual reporting procedures in this aspect of the practice of clinical child neuropsychology, this case also is presented in the quasi-report format used for the previous case (John). This format for the presentation of Bob's NLD-related neuropsychological test results—and especially that employed for the neuropsychological formulation and recommendations that appear toward the end of it—should be considered in light of the fact that litigation was pending in regard to a craniocerebral trauma that he had sustained as a toddler. Interested parties in such a situation (e.g., lawyers, parents) are most often quite concerned about the long-term prognosis for a child so afflicted, especially with regard to academic, vocational, and social pursuits.

Background

Bob was referred at the age of 6 years, 8 months for neuropsychological assessment in order to determine the nature and extent of his adaptive skills and abilities. It was reported that, at the age of 16 months, he had sustained a compound depressed skull fracture of the right temporo-parietal region.

Behavioral Observations during the Examination

During the morning session of this examination, Bob was much more alert and cooperative than he was during the afternoon session. Throughout the examination, he was quite talkative. Overall, he exhibited an average level of general physical activity. For the most part, he was easily distracted, although reasonably attentive when closely supervised. On some occasions he was quite careless in carrying out tasks. There were also some instances when he became antagonistic toward the examiner. In general, he exhibited a rather low level of tolerance with frustration. On occasion his motivation to do well on the tasks administered was in some doubt. He often required encouragement to continue on tasks that he perceived as difficult. There were occasions when he seemed not to understand test instructions as fully as would be expected.

All things considered, it would appear that we obtained a reasonably reliable estimate of this boy's adaptive skills and abilities in this examination. It is clear, however, that we can have much more confidence in the reliability of his good performance than we can have in his poor performance.

Summary of Test Results and Impressions

Bob's test results are summarized in Figure 7.7. Although there was some doubt about the reliability of some of his levels of performance in this examination, there was enough information available from comparisons of performance on the two sides of the body and from other methods of test analysis to suggest strongly that the bulk of his current problems in adaptation are consistent with the expected long-term sequelae of a severe craniocerebral trauma maximally involving the temporo-parietal region of the right cerebral hemisphere. The prognosis for cognitive, social, and general adaptational recovery from such deficits is usually quite guarded. Indeed, our usual expectation is for children who have sustained such damage to experience increasing difficulties in a variety of areas as they grow older. The following are some of the specific problems.

Although Bob's test results showed no indications of any simple tactile imperception, there was evidence of marked tactile suppression with the left hand under conditions of bilateral simultaneous tactile stimulation of the left hand and the right side of the face. There was some evidence of finger agnosia and astereognosis for forms with the left hand.

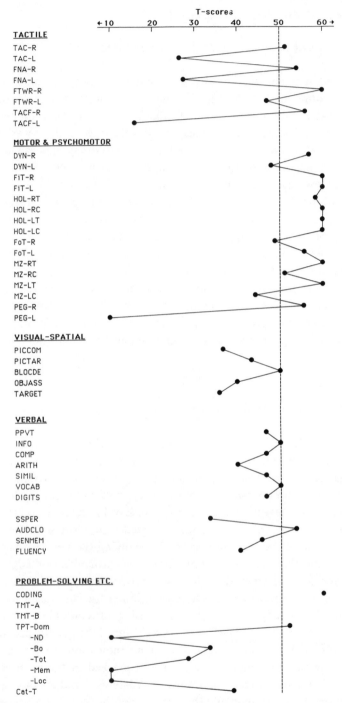

FIGURE 7.7. Summary of Bob's neuropsychological test results. (TMT-A and TMT-B were not administered.)

194

	Testing 1 (6 yr, 8 mo)
WISC-R	
VIQ	94
PIQ	92
FSIQ	92
Underlining (no. of each)	
Superior	0
Average	3
Borderline	1
Mild	7
Moderate	2
Severe	0
Speed subtest	Average
WRAT-R (grade; centile)	
Reading	1; 23
Spelling	<1; 5
Arithmetic	1; 21
PIC (*T* score)	
Lie	42
F	67
Defensiveness	56
Adjustment	66
Achievement	74
Intellectual Screening	76
Development	75
Somatic Concern	61
Depression	51
Family Relations	55
Delinquency	73
Withdrawal	43
Anxiety	61
Psychosis	54
Hyperactivity	62
Social Skills	66
ARS	
No	16
Little	11
Very much	3
BPC	
No	38
Little	26
Very much	2

FIGURE 7.7. (continued)

EXAMPLE FROM WRAT SPELLING SUBTEST

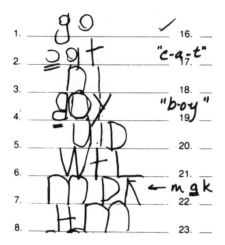

Bob also exhibited much more marked finger dysgraphesthesia with the left hand than with the right.

On the Tactual Performance Test he performed within normal limits when using the right hand; however, left-hand performance was severely impaired. There was no clear evidence that he was able to benefit from experience with this task.

There were no indications of any simple auditory imperception or suppression. Performance on a Sweep Hearing Test was negative.

He performed very poorly on the Rosner Auditory Analysis Test, a task requiring complex auditory analysis of common words. Performance on tests for sound-blending (Auditory Closure Test) and verbatim memory for sentences of gradually increasing length (Sentence Memory Test) was within normal limits. Bob performed below normal limits on a test designed for the measurement of phonemically cued verbal fluency and on the Speech-Sounds Perception Test. It is notable, however, that he became much more efficient on the latter task after considerable experience with it. This may reflect a more general aspect of his adaptive behavior, namely, easier adaptation to verbal than to nonverbal tasks.

On an Aphasia Screening Test there was no evidence of dysnomia or more than ordinary problems in simple arithmetic calculation. Although Bob did make some errors on some items of this test, there was no evidence of any frank aphasic deficits. It is notable that he misspelled his surname on two attempts during the test.

On the WISC-R Bob obtained a Verbal IQ of 94. Subtest scaled scores on this section ranged from a low of 7 on the Arithmetic subtest to highs of 10 on the Information and Vocabulary subtests. It is evident that this boy does not have more than age-appropriate difficulties with the more prosaic, rote aspects of verbal skills.

On the Peabody Picture Vocabulary Test, designed as a test of receptive vocabulary, he obtained a Mental Age of 6 years, 6 months, which is equivalent to an IQ of 95.

There were no indications of any simple visual imperception or suppression. He performed at a mildly to moderately impaired level on a task requiring immediate memory for visual sequences (Target Test).

Overall, Bob's performance on tests for various aspects of visual discrimination and visual-spatial-organizational skills was quite variable. He did well on one test involving visual discrimination and matching (Matching V's Test) and poorly on others (Matching Figures Test; Matching Pictures Test). He performed relatively well on some subtests of the Underlining Test and rather poorly on others. He had no difficulty with a task requiring him to alternate between form and shape to negotiate a visual-spatial array (Progressive Figures Test), but he encountered considerable problems when required to use shape and color alternately for this purpose (Color Forms Test). There is much in his performance on these types of "visual" tasks to indicate that his level of motivation was fluctuating, that he did not pay close attention to what he was doing, and that he was not inclined to persist in these tasks when they became difficult for him.

On the WISC-R he obtained a Performance IQ of 92. Subtest scaled scores on this section were quite variable, ranging from a low of 6 on the Picture Completion subtest to a high of 14 on the Coding subtest. A discrepancy in performance of this magnitude is difficult to explain solely on the basis of his presumably intact and deficient skills and abilities. Rather, it would appear that fluctuating motivation and attention may have been primarily responsible for the discrepancy in these results. At the same time, it is clear that these types of "visual" tasks are more likely to eventuate in this type of behavior than are tasks of a more verbal, rote, prosaic character.

Bob would appear to be exclusively right-handed and right-footed. Eye dominance appeared mixed. Strength of grip with the right hand was well above normal limits; that with the left, within normal limits. Finger-tapping speeds were superior bilaterally. Foot-tapping speeds were approximately normal bilaterally. There were no indications of any static or kinetic tremor on tests designed specifically for the measurement of these dimensions of motor skill. Performance on a speeded eye–hand coordination task (Grooved Pegboard Test) was average with the right hand and severely impaired with the left hand. It is apparent that this boy's problems in the use of the left hand increase dramatically as the requirements for the coordination of various sorts of input (e.g., visual, tactile) in the carrying out of the psychomotor task increase.

His graphic renderings of simple visual designs were approximately age appropriate, with no evidence of any gross visual-spatial distortions in them. There were some instances of reversals in his printing of some letters. His printing was approximately age appropriate.

On the Category Test his overall level of performance was mildly impaired. (The younger children's version of this test is *not* a hypothesis-testing or concept-formation task; rather, it appears to have a very different factorial structure than the older children's version.)

On the WRAT-R he obtained the following approximate grade-equivalents and centile scores, respectively: Reading, 1(23); Spelling, <1(5); and Arithmetic, 1(21). On the Spelling subtest there was clear evidence of an emerging capacity to appreciate the phonemic aspects of words. His approach to the reading of unfamiliar words was of the "best-guess/sight-word" variety, which led him to guess *jump* for *jar*, *over* for *even*, *there* for *then*, and so forth. He was capable of simple addition on the Arithmetic subtest.

The mother and father each completed the Personality Inventory for Children independently. In neither case was the perceived level of socio-emotional functioning of this boy within the pathological range. The father's responses on rating scales for hyperactivity and common behavior problems were also not within the range of significant psychopathology. Those items that were endorsed would seem to suggest that Bob is perceived as somewhat difficult to handle in some situations and that he is somewhat prone to excessive activity in some instances.

Although clearly not diagnostic of any neuropathological condition, this particular pattern of neuropsychological test results would be compatible with the expected long-term sequelae of a significant craniocerebral trauma that has maximally affected the functional integrity of the middle (temporal-parietal) regions of the right cerebral hemisphere. Functions ordinarily thought to be subserved primarily by the more anterior and posterior regions of the right cerebral hemisphere appear to be largely intact. Indications of some deficits in selected aspects of psycholinguistic skills would be consistent with the expected contre-coup effects within the left cerebral hemisphere of the reported craniocerebral trauma; these deficits are relatively mild.

Prognosis and Recommendations

Significant lesions within the right cerebral hemisphere at an early age are often found to have long-lasting negative impact on personal, social, and vocational adaptation. The presence of relatively intact verbal skills often masks the nature of problem-solving and other deficiencies which tend to increase with the passing of time. This being the case, early intervention is very important in such cases. The following points relate to specific aspects of prognosis and intervention for this boy.

It is my distinct impression that Bob will probably exhibit the academic, social, and vocational deficits that are expected to characterize the "NLD child." My best estimate is that he would be expected to suffer a moderate degree of deficiency within these areas of adaptive functioning.

With respect to this boy's academic status, I would predict that he would be most likely to benefit from methods of teaching that are primarily verbal in nature. He would also be expected to do reasonably well in areas of educational content that are primarily verbal in nature, that can be studied and learned in a rote fashion, and that depend primarily upon verbal memory for the demonstration of levels of learning. He would be expected to do quite poorly in areas such as mathematics and science. Indeed, he would be expected to perform least well in any academic area that places a premium upon concept formation, strategy generation, hypothesis testing, and adaptive problem solving. These difficulties are expected to become more prominent and evident as he develops.

With respect to Bob's eventual vocational status, the same principles enunciated in the previous paragraph would be expected to obtain. That is, I would predict that he would do well in vocations that require verbal input and output for communication, that are programatic in nature, and that place a premium upon verbal memory. He would be expected to do poorly at vocations that demand much in the way of trouble shooting, complex eye–hand coordination, and flexible and adaptive behavior in novel situations.

Intervention will probably be required for the duration of his years in school and for some time thereafter. (The treatment regimen that I would recommend for this boy is outlined in the last part of this chapter.) During the school years, the cost of such intervention would probably be minimal because much of it could be provided by the special services capabilities that most school systems possess. At the same time, it would be well to have a neuropsychological consultant who is close to the situation and who could be called upon to advise Bob's academic caretakers of appropriate modifications in programing for him. Such a consultant should also be available to his parents, since treatment for such individuals must involve virtually every venue of their adaptive functioning.

Bob's needs for intervention following the school years are very difficult to estimate. Much depends upon how well he has progressed to that point. It is abundantly clear, however, that individuals who suffer from the deficiencies that are currently evident in this boy tend to need much in the way of support and active intervention in their adult years. In my experience, this support and intervention are usually provided by various types of vocational–rehabilitation services and mental health professionals.

Again, family cooperation and collaboration in the treatment program are integral aspects of intervention for children such as this. Although time off from work on the part of the parents may not be required to effect this program, it is usually the case that much extra time (as compared to that required for "normal" children) is needed for interaction with such a child. This is occasioned by their needs for repetition, practice, and step-by-step monitoring when engaged in novel tasks.

In general, the effects of significant right-hemisphere damage are thought to have an increasingly impairing effect upon adaptive behavior during the course of development. Although this scenario is not inevitable, it appears with sufficient frequency to render it highly probable. Given this probability, it is crucial that intervention begin as early as possible following such an insult.

The practical implications and ramifications of our neuropsychological findings for Bob with respect to higher education, employment, and physical skills have been described in a general way. More specifically, it would be well to assess these on an ongoing basis. I assert this because it is probable that treatment at this time would serve to mitigate and mollify somewhat many of the usually very negative long-term consequences that so often plague individuals afflicted early in development by this type of symptom complex. There is no guarantee, however, that such will be the case. Indeed, we are usually satisfied to see that such individuals do not become increasingly worse during the course of intervention.

I would recommend that a repeat comprehensive neuropsychological assessment be carried out on this boy approximately 1 year after this initial assessment. This would afford the opportunity to assess his progress over this crucial developmental time span, and it would also allow for a determination of any rehabilitational needs that should be addressed specifically within the academic situation, just before he begins another year at school.

In order to determine the reversibility of Bob's current condition, it will be necessary to follow him for some time. As already pointed out, I am not disposed to be sanguine about the possibilities for permanent recovery from such deficits. At the same time, it is prudent to allow the facts to speak for themselves.

PROGNOSIS AND GENERAL TREATMENT PROGRAM FOR NLD PATIENTS

With these case illustrations as background, we turn now to a consideration of issues relating to prognosis and treatment for the NLD children and adolescents. These sections are couched in fairly broad terms, with an emphasis upon general principles. The reader would do well to consider the applicability of each of these principles and suggested practices to each of the cases that have been discussed to this point.

Prognosis

The findings of a study mentioned in Chapter 3 (Rourke, Young, et al., 1986) are relevant here. It was found that, of the eight NLD adults who were selected for study, seven had obtained some form of postsecondary school education. None of these persons, however, held jobs that were commensurate with their academic qualifications. All of them exhibited emotional and social difficulties and, in general, had a poor understanding of their adaptive limitations. Some of them had carried a diagnosis of schizophrenia at some point in their adult lives. In all cases, the prognosis for future adjustment and independent living, without the benefit of involvement from various social agencies, was viewed as quite guarded.

The findings of the Rourke, Young, et al. (1986) study of NLD adults should come as no surprise, in view of the particular pattern of neuropsychological strengths and deficiencies exhibited by NLD children. As we have seen throughout this book, these include difficulties in benefiting from nonverbal experiences and an unusual reliance on language as a primary tool for adaptation. There is also the confusion of their parents and other caretakers concerning the nature of significance of their condition, and the inappropriate expectations of such children by all concerned.

Although not all children who exhibit the NLD syndrome have identical developmental histories or behave exactly as outlined in this and the foregoing chapters, the similarities in behavioral outcomes for such children are remarkably similar. At the same time, it is clear that the ability of these children's primary caretakers to understand their deficiencies early in life and to generate appropriate expectations for them are important factors in determining the degree to which they will exhibit maladaptive or atypical behavior in later childhood. Furthermore, thoughtful parental guidance and specialized forms of treatment outside of the home situation are important determinants of general prognosis. Finally, the *degree* of neuropsychological impairment would appear to be a crucial consideration. Children whose abilities are extremely impaired and who exhibit the full constellation of neuropsychological difficulties that are the hallmarks of the NLD syndrome are those who would appear to be most at risk for maladaptive consequences.

Remediation and Habilitation

Outlined here are some common features of an integrated and carefully orchestrated program of intervention that we have found to be helpful for children and adolescents who exhibit the NLD syndrome. This material is an adapted and expanded version of that contained in Strang and Rourke (1985a); general considerations relating to the care and treatment of brain-impaired children and adolescents are outlined in Rourke, Bakker, et al. (1983, especially Chapter 6). The program involves the principal caretakers—parents, teachers, and therapists—at every step of the way. For example, one of the first steps in a remediation–habilitation program involves providing the parents with appropriate information concerning the nature and significance of their child's neuropsychological disabilities. Often the child's parents require ongoing counseling and support in order to gear their expectations and their parenting methods and techniques to fit the child's most salient developmental needs.

Remediation and habilitation for NLD children is crucial but difficult. Part of this difficulty relates to the impression that persists in the minds of many involved in the educational process that children who read and spell well could not possibly have any unusual educational needs. This being the case, such children are seldom involved in educational programs that are appropriate for their special learning needs. This is particularly unfortunate because, if treatment is not instituted fairly early on all fronts (including academic) in such a child's life, the prognosis tends to be quite bleak. With these remarks as background, the following general principles of intervention for principal caregivers are offered.

Observe Behavior

It is important to observe children's behavior closely, especially in novel or otherwise complex situations. Focus on what they do and disregard what they say. This should help the parents, therapists, and/or teachers to develop a better appreciation of each child's potentially outstanding adaptive deficiencies and to shape their own cognitive "set" for interventions with the child. One of the most frequent criticisms of remedial intervention programs with this particular type of child is that remedial authorities are unaware of the extent and significance of the child's deficiencies. Through direct observation it should become apparent that the child is very much in need of a systematic, well-orchestrated program of intervention.

Adopt a Realistic Attitude

Once it has been established that the child's behavior is nonadaptive, particularly in new or otherwise complex situations, one must then be realistic in assessing the import and impact of the child's neuropsychological strengths (e.g., "automatic" language skills, rote memory) and deficiencies (e.g., visual-spatial-organizational skills). In the classroom, for instance, it should be readily apparent that these children's well-developed word-recognition and spelling abilities are not sufficient for them to benefit from many forms of formal and informal instruction, especially for those subjects that require visual-spatial-organizational and/or non-verbal problem-solving skills. This being the case, there are really only two educational alternatives, either to adopt special procedures for the presentation of material of the latter variety or to avoid such material altogether.

Use a Systematic Approach

Teach these children in a systematic, step-by-step fashion. Whenever, possible, use a parts-to-whole verbal teaching approach. As a rule of thumb, therapists and teachers should take note that, if it is possible to talk about an idea, concept, or procedure in a straightforward fashion, then these children should be able to grasp at least some aspects of the material. On the other hand, if it is not possible to put into words an adequate description of the material to be learned (e.g., as in explaining time concepts), it will probably be quite difficult for NLD children to benefit from the instruction.

It should also be kept in mind that these children will learn best when each of the verbal "steps" is in the correct sequence, because of their inadequate problem-solving skills and associated organizational difficulties with novel (even linguistically novel) material. A secondary benefit of this teaching approach is that the children are provided with a set of verbal rules that can be written out and then reapplied whenever it is appropriate to do so. This is particularly important for the teaching of mechanical arithmetic operations and procedures.

The principal impediment to engaging in this rather slow and painstaking approach to teaching NLD children is the fact that caregivers often have the faulty impression that these children are much more adept and adaptable than is actually the case. This increases the probability of caregivers starting a program at a level that is too sophisticated and will proceed at too fast a clip for the information-processing capacities of these children. NLD children on the other hand, tend to respond quite appreciatively and appropriately to an approach that is slow, repetitive, and highly redundant.

Among the other specific educational recommendations for these children are the following: (1) teach and emphasize reading comprehension skills as soon as the children have gained a functional appreciation of sound–symbol correspondence; (2) institute regular handwriting drills early in the educational career, to help further development of these skills; (3) before proceeding with any copying task, teach children to read the material to be copied carefully; (4) teach children verbal strategies that will help them to organize written work; (5) teach mechanical arithmetic in a systematic, verbal, step-by-step fashion, as outlined in some detail in Strang and Rourke (1985b); and (6) involve the child as much as possible in skill-level-appropriate physical education experiences. With respect to the latter point, it should be borne in mind that motor learning of all sorts is difficult but necessary for NLD children. Indeed, since such children learn to decode words and spell at superior levels without any appreciable teaching or other assistance, it would be well to substitute various types of physical activities during times when word decoding and spelling are being taught to their classmates.

Cultivate Social Awareness

Encourage children to describe in detail important events that are transpiring in their lives. This remedial recommendation applies not only to teaching sessions but also to any situation in which children do not seem to appreciate fully the significance of their behavior or the behavior of others. For example, when there is an incident on the playground in which the child has encountered interpersonal difficulty, ask him/her to explain in detail the events that transpired and what he/she perceives to be the cause of the incident and its effects. Encourage the child to focus on the relevant aspects of the situation, and point out the irrelevancies that are brought up. Through discussion, help the child to become aware of discrepancies between his/her perceptions regarding the situation in question and the perceptions of others. In teaching situations, one technique found useful is to encourage children to "reteach" their teachers or therapists (or, in some situations, teach other children) the procedure or concept that they themselves have been taught. This will help to increase the probability that the children have understood the necessary information, that it has been analyzed and integrated, and that it will be applied in future situations.

Teach Specific Problem-Solving Strategies

Teach the children appropriate strategies for dealing with particularly troublesome situations that occur on a frequent, everyday basis. In many cases, NLD children do not generate appropriate problem-solving strategies independently because they are unaware of the actual requirements of the situation, or because this particular type of endeavor requires basic neuropsychological competencies that they have not developed. For both of these reasons, such children need to be taught appropriate strategies for handling the requirements of frequently occurring troublesome situations. The teacher or therapist will find that the step-by-step requirements for teaching NLD children are quite similar to those that would be employed effectively for much younger children. Once again, it should be emphasized that the most frequent error made by adult caretakers in such situations is to overestimate these children's capacities to learn and apply adaptive problem-solving solutions and techniques for coping.

Encourage Generalization of Learned Strategies and Concepts

Although the majority of "normal" children see how one particular strategy or procedure may apply to a number of different situations, and/or how certain concepts may apply to a wide range of topics, NLD children usually exhibit difficulties with this form of generalization. For example, it is common to find that, although these children have been trained assiduously in visual attention and visual tracking skills in the laboratory or therapeutic setting, they fail to employ the skills effectively in everyday life, such as when it would be propitious to examine some aspects of a person's physical characteristics in order to enhance recognition of that person in the future. It is abundantly clear that NLD children not only need to be taught specific skills in a step-by-step fashion, but also that transitional or generalization skills need to be addressed in an identical manner.

Improve Verbal Skills

Teach children to refine and use appropriately their verbal (expressive) skills. As has been pointed out previously, it is quite probable that they will come to use these skills much more frequently and for much different reasons than do most children. For example, they may repeatedly ask questions as a primary way of gathering information about a new or otherwise complex situation. This may be quite inappropriate for many situations, especially those of a social nature, in which nonverbal behaviors are much more important for feedback and direction.

The content of verbal responses may also be problematic. A common observation is that NLD children may begin to make a reply by directly addressing the question asked, but then gradually drift off into a completely different topic. At the very least, the tangential nature of such utterances has the effect of alienating the listener. Specific training should be undertaken that is directed at "what-to-say," "how-to-say," and "when-to-say" aspects of language, as these questions apply to the children's problem areas. As with other aspects of remediation, however, there is the problem of generalization of learning in this sort of training exercise. NLD children tend not to be flexible and adaptive in the application of learned habits, even when these are in their areas of strength (i.e., verbal skills).

Strengthen Development in Areas of Weakness

Teach children to make better use of their visual-perceptual-organizational skills. It should be borne in mind that children tend to "lead with their strong suit" in situations that are in any way problematic for them. For example, children who exhibit extreme disability in visual-spatial skills in combination with relatively intact receptive and expressive verbal skills tend to use the verbal skills whenever possible, even though it may be inappropriate to do so. This encourages a situation in which the poorly developed skills are not challenged or "exercised," so that optimal development may not be realized. The tendency to "play one's strong suit" also encourages children to develop other ways of using language-related skills, many of which are clearly maladaptive.

To increase the likelihood that children's visual modality and associated perceptive and analytic abilities will be developed and used optimally, younger children could be taught to name visual details in pictures as a way of encouraging them to pay attention to these details. In conjunction with this exercise, they could be asked to talk about the relationship between various details in a picture (e.g., intersecting lines) as a way of drawing attention to the complexity, importance, and significance of visual features of stimulus presentation.

With older children, remedial suggestions and exercises should be more "functional" or practical in nature but at the same time should address directly particular areas of great difficulty. For example, consider the fact that most social situations require children to decipher or decode the nonverbal behaviors of others in order to interpret them properly, an area in which NLD children are quite deficient. Therefore, one might create "artificial" social situations that require children to rely only on their visual-receptive and other nonverbal skills for interpretation. This could be done with pictures, films, or even contrived "real-life" situations for which there is no verbal feedback available. After an exercise of this type, one should discuss each child's perception of the social situation and of his or her most appropriate role in the situation. At the same time, one might provide the child with strategies for deciphering the most salient nonverbal dimensions inherent in these contrived social situations.

Aid Child in Interpretation of Competing Stimuli

Teach children to interpret visual information when there is "competing" auditory information. This type of training is usually more complex than the suggested remedial interventions already mentioned, but it is particularly important when attempting to teach children to deal more effectively with novel social situations. It is important not only to be able to interpret others' nonverbal behavior correctly but also to interpret what is being said in conjunction with these nonverbal cues. In most cases, this type of training should be undertaken only when there has been adequate work and progress in the previously mentioned areas.

Teach Appropriate Nonverbal Behavior

Many NLD children do not appear to have adequately developed nonverbal behavior. For example, such children often present with a somewhat "vacant" look or other inappropriate facial expressions. This is especially the case for those individuals who are found to exhibit marked neuropsychological deficits. Thus, for example, they may smile when they are experiencing failure with a task. It is important to attempt to teach more appropriate nonverbal behavior, keeping in mind the concepts introduced in association with the refinements of verbal expressive skills. In this connection, teaching children what to do and how and when to do it should be the focus of concern. For example, some children may not know how or when to convey their feelings in a nonverbal manner. Using informative pictures and imitative drills, working with a mirror, and other techniques and concrete aids can prove to be invaluable in this type of training. This sort of intervention may also serve to make children more aware of the significance of the nonverbal behavior of others.

Facilitate Structured Peer Interactions

It is not always possible to promote social training in unstructured social situations, because these are largely beyond the reach of the remedial therapist or teacher. For instance, when children are on the school playground, it is not often possible to regulate their play in any way, at least not to the extent that it promotes positive social growth for socially impaired youngsters. However, intramural activities of one sort or another, clubs, and formal community groups can provide a forum for social training if exploited in a proper manner. Unfortunately, because many children of this type tend to be somewhat socially withdrawn, they may not be encouraged to join their peers in social activities of any kind, as a "protective" maneuver on the part of parents and other caretakers. This attitude needs to be addressed and dealt with as early as possible in this remedial program.

Provide Structure for Exploration

Promote, encourage, and monitor "systematic" explorative activities. One of the most potentially harmful tacks that a well-meaning therapist can take with NLD children is to leave them to their own devices in activities that lack sufficient (or any) structure, such as ambient play situations with other children. On the other hand, it is quite worthwhile to design specific activities through which children are encouraged to explore their environment. For example, exploratory activity may be encouraged within the structure of a gross motor program. In this setting, children could be provided with the opportunity to explore various types of apparatus and the exercises that would suit each apparatus. It is important to insure that children do not feel as if they are competing with their peers. In addition, following the lesson, children should be required to give the instructor some verbal feedback and, perhaps, accompanying demonstrations regarding the activities that have transpired.

Give Instruction in the Use of Aids

Older children of at least 10 years of age can be taught how to use available aids to reach specific goals. One potential aid is a hand-held calculator, which can provide children with a way of checking the accuracy of their mechanical arithmetic work, after they have completed a question independently. (This, of course, is dependent on correct use of the calculator.) If it is found that the solution is incorrect, children should then be encouraged to rework the question with pencil and paper. At the high-school level, hand calculators should probably be used whenever possible, so that young adults will develop at least a functional grasp of common mathematical operations and their applications in everyday life situations.

Another aid that could be used, especially for younger children, is a digital watch. We have found that many such children have difficulty in reading the hands of a traditional type of watch, and that this imposes further limitations on their already impoverished appreciation of time concepts. A digital watch is more easily read and can serve as a concrete tool for the teaching of elementary time concepts.

In all of this, there is no substitute for creative approaches to the provision of therapeutic aids. This is especially the case for the exploitation of the vast potential of computers as prosthetic/therapeutic devices. Programs that allow for appropriate and helpful corrective feedback for difficult academic subjects; those that take children in a step-by-step fashion through any number of quasisocial and problem-solving situations; those that present material in a systematic, sequenced fashion that draws children's attention to the process of problem-solving development; and many more dimensions of the creative use of computer software are potentially of considerable benefit for NLD children and adolescents.

Encourage Accurate Self-Evaluation

Help children to gain insight into which situations are easy for them and which are potentially troublesome. It is important for older children and adolescents to gain a reasonably realistic view of their capabilities. This is certainly more easily said than done. In this regard, therapists' expectations always need to be in concert with the children's abilities, since gains in this area may prove to be marginal at best. For instance, it may be that a child's early practical insight may be limited to "I am good at spelling and have problems with math." However, if provided with consistent and appropriate feedback from concerned and informed adults regarding his/her performance in various kinds of situations, fairly sophisticated insights may develop. This is especially important with respect to perceiving the need to use prelearned strategies in appropriate situations. Furthermore, it is important that NLD children learn that they do have some cognitive strengths, which they can use to advantage in specific situations.

Work with All Caretakers

The efforts of all caretakers should be coordinated and supported, to keep them focused on the child's most salient developmental needs. All of the recommendations that have been made already can apply to the style and emphasis that caretakers could incorporate into their relations with NLD children. We have found that well-motivated caretakers who have an intuitive or learned appreciation of such children's adaptive strengths and weaknesses most often create a milieu at home or elsewhere in which the children prosper and in which adaptive deficiencies are minimized. Unfortunately, this ideal caretaker–child relationship is not often found; in consequence, it is usually necessary for concerned professionals to assume a major responsibility for guiding principal caretakers. In some cases, it may be advisable and/or necessary to employ highly structured "parenting" programs, such as Holland's (1983) Directive Parental Counseling, to assist various caretakers in the habilitational process.

Encourage Development of Life Skills

Be cognizant of the therapist's or remedial specialist's role in preparing NLD children for adult life. Special educators, in particular, should assume a major responsibility for this. Unlike most educational programs, in which the primary goal is to help children to master a particular curriculum, the program required by NLD children is one that focuses primarily on the development of life skills. These children's mastery of the standard academic curriculum is insignificant if they are not prepared to meet the social and other adaptive demands of independent living. Indeed, we have found through longitudinal follow-up that some NLD children as adults have developed rather seriously debilitating forms of psychopathology. This being the case, it is clear that remedial/habilitational interventions with such children should always be consonant with their short- and long-term remedial needs and capacities.

LIMITATIONS OF THE CURRENT MODEL

The NLD model proposed in Chapter 6 and illustrated with case presentations in the current chapter is meant to serve as a first approximation to several important components of a developmental neuropsychological theory that is capable of embracing what is currently known regarding ontogenetic changes in brain–behavior relationships, especially with regard to the impact and interactions of various forms of brain disease, disorder, and dysfunction on such development. It is, of course, also designed to serve a heuristic purpose vis-à-vis experimental tests of its propositions. At the same time, it should be borne in mind that there are several findings that do not fit precisely within this proposed theoretical framework at this time.

For example, it is known that approximately one-half of the published acallosal cases exhibit lower Verbal IQ than Performance IQ, while the other half exhibit the opposite pattern (Dennis, 1977). Also, Dennis (1981) has presented a very thorough analysis of the linguistic and visual-spatial skills of an 27-year-old adult who had complete agenesis of the corpus callosum (with a Dandy–Walker cyst in the posterior fossa), who obtained a Verbal IQ of 96, a Performance IQ of 119, and a Full Scale IQ of 106. While the results of the latter study, especially the absence of any apparent visual-spatial-organizational deficits, stand in marked contrast to those of Mary in this chapter and the general manifestations of the NLD syndrome, it should be remembered that Mary did not have any apparent cystic formation and that her acallosal status appeared to be relatively "pure" (i.e., not complicated by the presence of any other abnormal structure in the region that the corpus callosum is expected to occupy). Be that as it may, it is interesting to note that the acallosal adult described by Dennis (1981) exhibited a discrete loss of syntactic–pragmatic language function within the language domain, a characteristic that is quite typical of the NLD child.

As suggested earlier, it is expected that comprehensive investigations of more children and adolescents who present with significant white matter disease, disorder, and dysfunction will allow for a more precise specification of the components of the NLD model. Indeed, it is expected that many of the specific forms of neurological impairment, the effects of which this model is designed to embrace, will be shown to have their own unique features. Furthermore, it is expected that, even within these categories of neurological disease, there will emerge demonstrably unique subtypes, as has been shown by Dennis, Hendrick, Hoffman, and Humphreys (1987) in the case of hydrocephalic children and adolescents.

CONCLUSION

Our examination of the current formulation of the NLD syndrome and model is at an end, for now. There remains the task of honing the structure and dynamics of the syndrome and the model through the types of empirical research that were alluded to in Chapters 4, 5, and 6. Also, there is much need for the rigorous testing of the provisions of the treatment dimensions suggested in this chapter. Of central importance, from both a theoretical and clinical standpoint, is the investigation of the developmental manifestations of the NLD syndrome—whether these be complete, partial, or absent—in persons with demonstrable brain pathology. Of no less importance is the same quest in persons suffering from disorders wherein the neurological substrate is currently within the realm of hypothesis rather than established fact. My inclination is that investigations in the latter area (as, for example, were suggested in Chapter 6 with respect to autism) will turn out to be particularly fascinating, especially with regard to the "white matter hypothesis."

CHAPTER EIGHT

Implications for Learning Disability Definitions and Future Research

It may be of interest to situate the NLD syndrome within a broader context of research and theory in the neuropsychology of learning disabilities. This chapter constitutes an attempt to do so. No claim is made for the perspicacity of the formulations that follow. They are proffered as apparently plausible generalizations that fit with my review of the reasonably well-controlled studies that have appeared in the neuropsychological learning disability subtyping literature over the past 15 or so years. It is hoped that the following will serve some heuristic purposes, especially for those bold enough to test the propositions therein.

If there are reliable and valid differences between learning disability subtypes, and if we still wish to retain the term *learning disabilities* as a generic descriptor of this heterogeneous group of disorders, then there are at least two issues with which we must deal, as follows:

1. There is a need for generic definition. The current ones, of which an example will be given shortly, will probably do quite nicely. However, it might be well to focus the generic definition on the common content of this group of disorders, namely, difficulties in learning in one or more areas.
2. There is a need for specific definitions of specific subtypes. Some of these (e.g., NLD) can be formulated now. Others will need to wait upon further research.

GENERIC DEFINITION

The following modification of the National Joint Committee on Learning Disabilities (January 30, 1981) definition would appear appropriate:

Learning disabilities is a generic term that refers to a heterogeneous group of disorders manifested by significant difficulties in the mastery of one or more of the following: listening, speaking, reading, writing, reasoning, mathematical, and other skills and abilities that are traditionally referred to as "academic." The term *learning disabilities* is also appropriately applied in instances where persons exhibit significant difficulties in mastering social and other adaptive skills and abilities. In some cases, investigations of learning disabilities have yielded evidence that would be consistent with hypotheses relating central nervous system dysfunction to the disabilities in question. Even though a learning disability may occur concomitantly with other handicapping conditions (e.g., sensory impairment, mental retardation, social and emotional disturbance) or environmental influences (e.g., cultural differences, insufficient or inappropriate instruction, psychogenic factors), it is not the direct result of those conditions or influences. However, it is possible that emotional disturbances and other adaptive deficiencies may arise from the same patterns of central processing assets and deficits that generate the manifestations of academic and social learning disabilities. Learning disabilities may arise from genetic variations, biochemical factors, events in the pre- to perinatal period, or any other subsequent events resulting in neurological impairment.

SPECIFIC DEFINITIONS

All of the following subtypes are characterized in terms of the specific patterns of neuropsychological assets and deficits that are thought to be responsible for the particular manifestations of learning strengths and weaknesses exhibited by children within the subtype. Issues such as inadequate or inappropriate motivation or a mismatch between learning history and the specific demands of the academic environment are not dealt with. The emphasis is on the impact of the specific learning disability subtype on (1) academic learning in the elementary school years and (2) socioemotional adaptation. With the exception of NLD, these subtypal definitions have received very little investigative attention; they are more in the nature of hypotheses that could (and I think, should) be investigated.

In proposing the patterns of neuropsychological assets and deficits that characterize these hypothesized learning disability subtypes, reference will be made to Table 8.1. It contains a summary of group R-S characteristics and dynamics that is modeled after the description in Chapter 5 of the NLD syndrome and dynamics. (Readers also should refer to Figure 5.1, p. 87.) There would appear to be a few significant differences between group R-S and a group that we might refer to as group R-S-A (i.e., a group

TABLE 8.1. Summary of Group R-S Characteristics and Dynamics

	Assets	Deficits
Neuropsychological		
Primary	Tactile perception Visual perception Motor and psychomotor Novel material	Auditory perception
Secondary	Attention (tactile, visual) Exploratory behavior	Attention (auditory, verbal)
Tertiary	Memory (tactile, visual) Concept formation Problem solving	Memory (auditory, verbal)
Speech/language	Prosody Semantics > phonology Content Pragmatics Function?	Phonology Verbal reception Verbal repetition Verbal storage Verbal association Verbal output (volume)
Academic	Reading comprehension (late) Mathematics Science	Graphomotor Word decoding Reading comprehension (early) Spelling Verbatim memory Mechanical arithmetic
Socioemotional/ adaptational	Adaptation to novelty Social competence Emotional stability Activity level	???

characterized by outstandingly poor reading, spelling, *and* arithmetic). Reference to our earlier studies of group R-S-A (Group 1 in Rourke & Finlayson, 1978; Rourke & Strang, 1978) will confirm this view. The following discussion will focus on three major categories of learning disabilities: those characterized primarily by disorders of linguistic functioning, those manifest mainly in disorders of nonverbal functioning, and those where output functioning is impaired in all areas.

Linguistic Disorders

Basic Phonological Processing Disorder (BPPD)

Table 8.1 contains a description of this subtype. The following is a summary of the assets and deficits that characterize it:

1. *Neuropsychological assets.* Tactile-perceptual, visual-spatial-organizational, psychomotor, and nonverbal problem-solving and concept-formation skills and abilities are developed to an average to above-average degree. The capacity to deal with novelty and the amount and quality of exploratory behavior are average. Attention to tactile and visual input is normal.

2. *Neuropsychological deficits.* Disordered phonemic hearing, segmenting, and blending are paramount. Attention to and memory for auditory-verbal material are clearly impaired. Poor verbal reception, repetition, and storage are evident. The amount and quality of verbal associations are clearly underdeveloped; there is less than average amount of verbal output.

3. *Prognoses.*

a. *Academic.* Reading and spelling are affected, as are those aspects of arithmetic performance that require reading and writing. The symbolic aspects of writing are affected. The nonverbal aspects of arithmetic and mathematics are left unaffected. The prognosis for advances in reading and spelling and the verbal-symbolic aspects of writing and arithmetic must be very guarded.

b. *Socioemotional.* Socioemotional disturbance may occur if parents, teachers, and other caretakers establish unattainable goals for the child and/or if antisocial models and lifestyles hold reinforcing properties for the child that the school and other caretakers are unable to counteract. When psychopathology occurs, it is likely to be of the acting-out variety. Another possibility is mild anxiety or depression.

Phoneme–Grapheme Matching Disorder (PGMD)

With reference to Table 8.1 and the description of the BPPD subtype, the following assets, deficits, and prognoses appear to apply:

1. *Neuropsychological assets.* Identical to BPPD subtype, except that phonemic hearing, segmenting, and blending are normal.

2. *Neuropsychological deficits.* Phoneme–grapheme matching problems are paramount, most often noticed in difficulties with translating graphemes to phonemes.

3. *Prognoses.*

a. *Academic.* Written spelling of "sight"-words may be average or better; written spelling of words not known "by sight" is as poor as in the BPPD subtype. Word-recognition is much better than that exhibited by the BPPD subtype, although still at an impaired level. Word-decoding skills may be as poor as for the BPPD subtype. Arithmetic and mathematics performance may rise to average or above-average levels when the words used in problems are minimized or learned "by sight." The prognosis for advances in reading and spelling is fair, much better than that for the BPPD subtype. Prognoses for advancement in arithmetic and mathematics are good, under the conditions just mentioned. Writing of unfamiliar words continues to be problematic.

b. *Socioemotional.* The prognosis for socioemotional disturbance is the same as that for the BPPD subtype, but with somewhat less risk.

Word-Finding Disorder (WFD)

This subtype is characterized by extreme problems in word-finding and verbal-expressive skills, within a context of a wide range of intact neuropsychological skills and abilities.

1. *Neuropsychological assets.* These are identical to those of the PGMD subtype, except that phoneme–grapheme matching skills are intact.

2. *Neuropsychological deficits.* The only major deficit is difficulty in accessing their normal store of verbal associations.

3. *Prognoses.*

a. *Academic.* Reading and spelling are very poor during early school years, with near-average or average performance in these areas emerging toward the end of the elementary school period (i.e., at approximately Grade 6 to 8). Arithmetic and mathematics are seen as early strengths. Writing of words that can be expressed and writing from a model are average to good.

b. *Socioemotional.* Prognosis for socioemotional functioning is virtually normal, but with the added minor risk factor of early failure in school.

Nonverbal Disorders: The NLD Syndrome

See Chapters 4 through 7 for a characterization of (1) the neuropsychological assets and deficits of this subtype of learning-disabled child and (2) the prognostic significance of these assets and deficits for academic and socioemotional functioning.

Output Disorders in All Modalities (OD)

This subtype is similar to the WFD subtype with respect to neuropsychological assets and deficits. Within the academic realm, there are the added problems of deficient output in the writing of words and written arithmetic.

1. *Neuropsychological assets.* Identical to WFD subtype.

2. *Neuropsychological deficits.* Identical to WFD subtype, with the additional difficulty of organizing, directing, and orchestrating all aspects of behavioral expression.

3. *Prognoses.*

a. *Academic.* Rather severe problems in oral and written output are prominent in early school years. Marked advances in word recognition, word decoding, and reading comprehension are evident in the middle school years. Written work remains poor, as does the capacity to deliver verbal descriptions and answers to questions.

b. *Socioemotional.* Such children are often characterized as having "acting-out" disorders in early school years. They are also at risk for social withdrawal and depression. This may develop into full-blown externalized and/or internalized forms of psychopathology, if management by the child's principal caretakers is inappropriate.

NEUROPSYCHOLOGICAL HYPOTHESES REGARDING SUBTYPES

The following hypotheses take the form of pointing to particular regions of the brain that are thought to be dysfunctional in the learning-disability subtypes that have been described. It should be emphasized that these hypotheses are meant to apply to the "developmental" presentation of learning disabilities and that they are thought to characterize these children's neuropsychological makeup since their earliest years. However, for a variety of reasons, such hypotheses are probably not currently testable until a child reaches the age of 9 or 10 years.

Linguistic Disorders

1. *Basic phonological processing disorder.* The locus of dysfunction is the secondary region of the temporal lobe of the left cerebral hemisphere.

2. *Phoneme–grapheme matching disorder.* The locus of dysfunction is the parieto-temporal (tertiary) region of the left cerebral hemisphere.
3. *Word-finding disorder.* The locus of dysfunction is the postero-inferior regions of the frontal lobe of the left cerebral hemisphere.

Nonverbal Disorders: The NLD Syndrome

The cause of this syndrome is disease, disorder, or dysfunction of the right cerebral hemisphere and/or diffuse white matter disease. White matter disturbance is primarily of interhemispheric or ascending fibers; significant associational fiber disturbance confined to the right hemisphere can also result in this disorder.

Output Disorders in All Modalities (OD)

The locus of this disorder is disturbance of function of the prefrontal regions of one or both cerebral hemispheres.

Notes

1. It is possible that a child may have more than one subtype of learning disability as a result of more than one location of brain dysfunction.

2. Very early insults to the brain that result in severe circumscribed focal dysfunction may be compensated for by the brain's limited capacities for reorganization and "plasticity." For these and many other reasons, the presence of a lesion in a particular region of the brain does not necessarily result in a learning disability of a particular subtype.

3. It would appear worthwhile to investigate the manifestations of learning disabilities in persons with various forms of (a) neurological disease, disorder, and dysfunction; (b) mental retardation; (c) socioemotional disturbance; (d) multilingualism; and (e) other forms of disturbance or difference that have been "traditionally" excluded from such study.

4. In each of the disorders mentioned in item 3, it is possible that one of the following scenarios would obtain:

a. The disorder (e.g., neurological disease, socioemotional disturbance) is present, but there are no associated central processing deficiencies. Thus, although the child may experience some *problems* in learning, there is no "learning disability" in evidence.

b. The disorder *plus* a learning disability are present, but there is no etiological connection between the disorder and the learning disability. For example, a child may have demonstrable neurological dysfunction or socioemotional disturbance that may or may not lead to learning problems, but the learning disability in evidence results from central processing deficiencies that are unrelated to the demonstrable neurological dysfunction or socioemotional disturbance.

c. The disorder is present and causes the learning disability. For example, phonemic hearing or visual-spatial-organizational deficiencies may be direct (i.e., primary) reflections of a particular type of neurological disease, and these deficiencies can be shown to lead directly to a particular subtype of learning disability.

d. Particular patterns of central processing assets and deficits may simultaneously eventuate in a particular subtype of learning disability and lead to a particular disorder (e.g., socioemotional disturbance).

5. It is possible that a general attentional deficit may interfere with academic and social learning. There is no reliable evidence to suggest that children with even rather marked degrees of attentional deficit need necessarily have any central processing deficiencies that would result in any subtypes of learning disability. General attentional deficits may coexist with modality-specific attentional deficiencies.

6. The visual–spatial subtype of disabled reader is almost always found at the very elementary grade school level. Evidence from a variety of sources suggests that this is an essentially transitory developmental phenomenon (i.e., a developmental lag). Children who exhibit such difficulties almost always make dramatic advances in reading and other aspects of academic learning with the passage of time. In this connection, it should be borne in mind that children who exhibit the NLD syndrome may be seen as "disabled readers" or at risk for reading disability early in their academic careers. However, the fact that they have outstanding visual-perceptual difficulties that persist into adulthood does not deter them from developing excellent word-recognition and word-decoding skills.

7. The contributions of right-hemisphere systems to various stages of word-decoding and reading comprehension are outlined in Chapter 4. Material in Chapters 4, 5, and 6 was designed to relate quite specifically to the broader roles of right-hemisphere systems and white matter functioning in all aspects of learning development and disability.

CONCLUSION

Finally, it should be emphasized that the material contained in this chapter is a mixture of some fairly well-established facts, some generalizations that appear plausible, and some purely hypothetical formulations. I view the principal merits of this exercise as heuristic; that is, I would hope that the generalizations and hypotheses that are explicated and nascent in the foregoing will be subject to creative empirical test. Indeed, I would be very pleased if the principal result of the formulations that lie at the heart of this book would be to encourage empirical examination and test of the elements of the NLD syndrome and model. It is certainly my intention to do so, and I would hope that others will be inclined to do likewise.

Descriptions of Tests Administered to Children (5–15 Years)

TESTS ADMINISTERED TO ALL CHILDREN (AGES 5–15)

Wechsler Intelligence Scale for Children (Wechsler, 1949)

Full Scale IQ. A composite score derived from the total scaled subtest scores. Indicative of overall "intellectual" functioning.

Verbal IQ. A prorated score derived from the total scaled scores of six Verbal subtests. Indicative of overall "verbal" functioning.

Performance IQ. A composite score derived from the scaled scores of the five Performance subtests (excluding the Mazes subtest). Indicative of overall nonverbal, "visual-perceptual" functioning.

Verbal Subtests

Information. Thirty questions. Involves elementary factual knowledge of history, geography, current events, literature, and general science. *Score*: number of items correct. *Task requirement*: retrieval of acquired verbal information. *Stimulus*: spoken question of fact. *Response*: spoken answer.

Comprehension. Fourteen questions. Involves the ability to evaluate certain social and practical situations. *Score*: number of items correct. *Task requirement*: evaluation of verbally formulated problem situations. *Stimulus*: spoken request for opinion. *Response*: spoken answer.

Arithmetic. Sixteen arithmetic problems of increasing difficulty. *Score*: number of problems correctly solved, within time credit. *Task requirement*:

arithmetic reasoning. *Stimulus*: spoken (first 13 items) or printed (last 3 items) question. *Response*: spoken answer.

Similarities. Sixteen pairs of words. The most essential semantically common characteristic of word pairs must be stated. *Score*: number correct. *Task requirement*: verbal abstraction. *Stimulus*: spoken question. *Response*: spoken answer.

Vocabulary. Forty words. Spoken definition of words. *Score*: number of words correct. *Task requirement*: verbal definition. *Stimulus*: spoken word. *Response*: spoken definition.

Digit Span. Repetition in forward order of three- to nine-digit numbers and repetition in reversed order of two- to eight-digit numbers. *Score*: simple total of forward and reversed digit span. *Task requirement*: short-term memory for digits. *Stimulus*: spoken numbers. *Response*: spoken numbers.

Performance Subtests

Picture Completion. Twenty pictures of familiar objects, each with a part missing. The missing part is identified from simple line drawings. *Score*: number of missing parts correctly identified. *Task requirement*: location of missing part on the basis of memory of the whole object. *Stimulus*: picture. *Response*: spoken name of missing part.

Picture Arrangement. Eleven series of picture cards. Pictures are sequentially arranged to form a story. *Score*: total credits for speed and accuracy of arrangement. *Task requirement*: manipulation of the order of picture cards to form the most probable sequence of events. *Stimulus*: pictures. *Response*: simple motor manipulation.

Block Design. Ten designs. Arrangement of colored blocks to form designs which match those on printed cards. *Score*: total score for speed and accuracy of block placement. *Task requirement*: arrangement of blocks to match a printed design. *Stimulus*: printed geometric design. *Response*: manipulation and arrangement of blocks.

Object Assembly. Four formboards (puzzles). Parts of each formboard are to be arranged to form a picture. *Score*: total score for speed and accuracy of assembly. *Task requirement*: spatial arrangement of parts to form a meaningful whole. *Stimulus*: disarranged parts of picture. *Response*: complex manipulation and arrangement of parts.

Coding. Ninety-three digits, preceded by a code which relates digits to symbols. Symbols are to be written below digits as rapidly as possible. *Score*:

number of symbols correctly written within a fixed time. *Task requirement*: association of digits and symbols by direct visual identification and/or by short-term memorization. *Stimulus*: printed digits and symbols. *Response*: rapid coordination of visual identification with a complex writing response. (For children under 8 years, symbols within common shapes are used; the score is the number of symbols correctly written in 45 shapes within a fixed time.)

Peabody Picture Vocabulary Test, Form A (Dunn, 1965)

Picture Vocabulary, Oral Raw Score, Oral IQ, Mental Age derived from IQ. One hundred fifty sets of four line drawings, with which 150 words of increasing difficulty are to be associated. The words are those of Form A of the Peabody Vocabulary Test. *Score*: total correct picture–word associations. *Task requirement*: selection of picture most appropriately related to the spoken word. *Stimulus*: four visual pictures, one spoken word. *Response*: simple pointing or verbal response. Oral IQ is the transformation of the oral raw score to an IQ score on the basis of test norms.

Wide Range Achievement Test (Jastak & Jastak, 1965)

Reading. Standardized test of oral word-reading achievement. *Score*: centile score based on total number of words correctly read aloud. *Task requirement*: association of printed letters with spoken word. *Stimulus*: printed word. *Response*: spoken word.

Spelling. Standardized test of written spelling achievement. *Score*: centile score based on total number of words correctly spelled. *Task requirement*: written production of spoken word. *Stimulus*: spoken word. *Response*: written word.

Arithmetic. Standardized test of written arithmetic achievement. *Score*: centile score based on total number of correct solutions to progressively more difficult arithmetic problems. *Task requirement*: solution of arithmetic problems. *Response*: written answers.

Personality Inventory for Children (Wirt, Lachar, Klinedinst, & Seat, 1977)

The Personality Inventory for Children (PIC) is an empirically and rationally constructed instrument that seeks to provide comprehensive and clinically relevant personality descriptions of individuals primarily in the range of 6–16 years of age. It is composed of 600 true–false questions regarding the child's behavior, disposition, interpersonal relations, and attitudes, and is to be completed by one of the child's parents.

The PIC contains 33 scales. Of these 33 scales, there are 16 profile scales and 15 supplementary scales. The PIC profile includes all scales judged to be most important. The PIC profile scales can be divided further into three validity scales (the Lie, F, and Defensiveness scales), one screening scale for general maladjustment (the Adjustment scale), and 12 clinical scales. The clinical scales include the following: Achievement; Intellectual Screening; Development; Somatic Concern; Depression; Family Relations; Delinquency; Withdrawal; Anxiety; Psychosis; Hyperactivity; and Social Skills. Score elevations in the positive direction (e.g., > 70 T) increase the likelihood of significant pathology for each of these scales.

OLDER CHILDREN'S BATTERY (AGES 9–15)

Tests for Sensory-Perceptual Disturbances (Reitan & Davison, 1974)

Tactile Perception

The child is required to identify correctly (without vision) the hand or face (left or right) which receives tactile stimulation. The stimulus is produced by a light touch. Following this determination of the child's ability to perceive unilateral stimulation, simultaneous bilateral hand stimulation and contralateral hand–face stimulation are interspersed with unilateral stimulation. The score is the number of errors for each hand and each side of the face under all conditions.

Auditory Perception

The child is required to identify correctly (without vision) the ear to which an auditory stimulus is presented. The stimulus is produced by rubbing the fingers together lightly. Following this determination of the child's ability to perceive unilateral stimulation, bilateral stimulation is interspersed with the unilateral stimulation. The score is the number of errors for each ear under all conditions.

Visual Perception

The child is required to identify correctly slight finger movements presented in a confrontation manner to the visual fields. Stimulation is presented first unilaterally and then simultaneous bilateral stimulation is interspersed with the unilateral trails. The score is the number of errors made within the quadrants of the visual fields.

Finger Agnosia

The child is required to identify (without the aid of vision) the finger which has been touched. Each of the five fingers is stimulated four times in a random order. First the right hand and then the left hand is stimulated. The score is the number of errors made with each finger for each hand.

Fingertip Number-Writing Perception

The child is required to verbalize (without the aid of vision) which of the numbers 3, 4, 5, or 6 has been written on his/her fingertips. A different finger of the right hand is used for each trial until four trials have been given for each finger. The procedure is then repeated for the left hand. The score is the number of errors made with each finger for each hand.

Coin Recognition

The child is required to identify, by tactile perception only, 1-, 5-, and 10-cent pieces placed in his/her right hand, then his/her left hand, and then each coin placed simultaneously in both hands. The order of presentation is unsystematic. The score is the number of errors made with each hand under each condition.

Target Test (Reitan & Davison, 1974)

The child is required to make a delayed response in reproducing visual-spatial configurations of increasing complexity tapped out by the examiner. The score is the number of items out of 20 correctly reproduced.

Trail Making Test (Reitan & Davison, 1974; Rourke & Finlayson, 1975)

The Trail Making Test consists of two parts, A and B. In A, the child is required, under time pressure, to connect the numbers 1 to 15 arranged on a page. The requirements are essentially similar in Part B, except that it is necessary to alternate between the numeric and the alphabetic series. The scores recorded are the number of seconds required to finish each part; the number of errors made on each part is also recorded.

Sweep Hearing Test

The child is required to indicate whether or not he/she can detect a series of pure tones, ranging from 125 Hz to 8,000 Hz. Each tone is presented unilaterally through ear phones. The decibel level of each tone is systematically decreased until the minimal audible level is determined.

Auditory Closure Test (Kass, 1964)

The child is required to blend into words 23 progressively longer chains of sound elements presented on tape. The score is the number of words correctly identified.

Sentence Memory Test (Benton, 1965)

The child is required to repeat sentences of gradually increasing length (from 1 to 26 syllables). These are presented on a tape recorder. The score is the number of sentences correctly repeated.

Speech-Sounds Perception Test (Reitan & Davison, 1974)

The child is required to attend to 30 tape-recorded nonsense syllables and to select the correct response alternative from among three printed choices. The score is the number of sounds correctly identified.

Verbal Fluency Test

The child is required to name as many words as he/she can, within 60 seconds, which begin with the sound "P," as in "pig." This is repeated with the sound "C," as in "cake." The score is the mean number of correct words for the two trials.

Auditory Analysis Test (Rosner & Simon, 1970)

The child is required to repeat a word and then repeat the same word with specific parts of it omitted. There are 40 progressively more difficult test items. The score is the total number of (modified) "words" correctly repeated.

Halstead–Wepman Aphasia Screening Test (Reitan & Davison, 1974)

Naming (*Dysnomia*). Five items which require the child to name familiar objects. *Score*: number of errors.

Spelling (*Spelling Dyspraxia*). The child is required to spell orally three spoken words. *Score*: number of errors.

Writing (*Dysgraphia*). Two items. The child is required to write a word and a sentence which are presented to him/her orally. *Score*: number of errors.

Enunciation (*Dysarthria*). Three items. The child is required to repeat three increasingly complex words spoken to him/her by the examiner. *Score*: number of errors.

Reading (*Dyslexia*). Six items. The child is required to read numbers, letters, and words. *Score*: number of errors.

Reproduction of Geometric Forms (*Constructional Dyspraxia*). Four items. The child is required to copy a square, a triangle, a Greek cross, and a key. *Score*: number of errors.

Arithmetic (*Dyscalculia*). Two items. The child is required to solve two problems: one subtraction (written) and one multiplication (oral). *Score*: number of errors.

Understanding Verbal Instructions (*Auditory–Verbal Agnosia*). Four items. The child is required to demonstrate an understanding of four verbal items. *Score*: number of errors.

Seashore Rhythm Test (Reitan & Davison, 1974)

The Rhythm Test is a subtest of the Seashore Tests of Musical Talent. The child is required to differentiate between 30 pairs of rhythmic patterns which are sometimes the same and sometimes different. The score is the number of errors.

Halstead Category Test (Reitan & Davison, 1974)

This test consists of 168 visual-choice stimulus figures which are presented to the child individually on a milk-glass screen located on the front of the apparatus. An answer panel is provided for the child. This consists of four answer buttons which are individually identified by the numbers 1, 2, 3, and 4. The child's task is to view the stimulus figure and to offer his/her answer by depressing one of the four answer buttons. A pleasant bell sounds after each correct response and a harsh buzzer sounds after each incorrect response. The bell and buzzer, therefore, provide the essential information necessary for determining the concept underlying the stimulus figures. In successive sequences of trials, the abstraction of principles of numerosity, oddity, spatial position, and relative extent is required for successful responding. The final subtest of the Category Test is of a summary nature and therefore does not have a principle to be discerned. The child is told to try to remember the correct answer based on his/her previous observation of the item and to give that same answer again. The score is the number of errors.

Tests for Lateral Dominance (Harris, 1947; Miles, 1929)

Hand Preference

The child is required to demonstrate the hand used to throw a ball, hammer a nail, cut with a knife, turn a doorknob, use scissors, use an eraser, and write his/her name. The number of tasks performed with each hand is recorded.

Eye Preference

The child is required to demonstrate the manner in which he/she would look through a telescope and use a rifle. The eye used for each task is recorded. In addition, the subject is given the Miles ABC Test for Ocular Dominance, in which (without ordinarily being aware of it) he/she has to choose one eye or the other to look through a conical apparatus to identify a visual stimulus. The eye chosen on each of 10 trials is recorded.

Foot Preference

The child is asked to demonstrate the manner in which he/she would kick a football and step on a bug. The foot used on each trial is recorded.

Strength of Grip (Reitan & Davison, 1974)

The Smedley Hand Dynamometer is used to measure strength of grip. The child is required to squeeze the dynamometer three times with the dominant hand and three times with the nondominant hand, alternating between hands on each trial. The mean pressure which the hand exerts on the three trials is recorded (in kilograms) for each hand.

Writing Speed (Reitan & Davison, 1974)

The child is required to write his/her name with a pencil as rapidly as possible, first with the preferred hand and then with the nonpreferred hand. The score is the time taken for each hand.

Finger Tapping (Reitan & Davison, 1974); Foot Tapping (Knights & Moule, 1967)

For finger tapping, the child uses alternately the index finger of the dominant hand and of the nondominant hand. Four trials of 10 seconds each are given for both hands. The Foot Tapping Test employs the same principles and instructions, but this time the child uses his/her feet, alternating between the dominant foot and the nondominant foot. Four trials of 10 seconds are given for each foot. The score for both finger and foot tapping is the average of the best three out of four trials.

Maze Test (Klove, 1963; Knights & Moule, 1968; Rourke & Telegdy, 1971)

The child is required to run a stylus through a maze which has the blind alleys filled and is placed at a 70° angle (on the Tactual Performance Test stand). Three scores are obtained: the number of contacts with the side of the maze, the total amount of time during which the stylus contacts the side of the maze, and the speed (total time from start to finish). These are electrically recorded. There are two successive trials with each hand. The scores are the totals for the two trials with the dominant hand and the two trials with the nondominant hand.

Graduated Holes Test (Klove, 1963; Knights & Moule, 1968; Rourke & Telegdy, 1971)

The child is required to fit a stylus into a series of progressively smaller holes. The idea is to hold the stylus in the center of the holes for a 10-second period without contacting the edge. Two scores are obtained: the number of contacts with the edge of the hole, and the duration of the contact. These are recorded electrically. The test is performed once with the right hand and once with the left hand.

Grooved Pegboard Test (Klove, 1963; Knights & Moule, 1968; Rourke, Yanni, MacDonald, & Young, 1973)

The child is required to fit keyhole-shaped pegs into similarly shaped holes on a 4″ × 4″ board beginning at the left side with the right hand and at the right side with the left hand. The child is urged to fit all 25 pegs in as rapidly as possible. One trial is performed with the dominant hand followed by one trial with the nondominant hand. The scores obtained are the length of time required to complete the task with each hand and the total number of times the pegs are dropped with each hand.

Tactual Performance Test (Reitan & Davison, 1974)

This test is Reitan's modification for children of the test developed by Halstead (1947). Halstead's test was based, in turn, upon a modification of the Seguin–Goddard formboard. The child is blindfolded and not permitted to see the formboard or blocks at any time. The formboard is placed in a vertical disposition at an angle of 70° on a stand situated on a table immediately in front of the child. He/she is to fit six blocks into the proper spaces with the dominant hand, then with the nondominant hand, and a third time using both hands. After the board and blocks have been put out of sight, the blindfold is removed and the child is required to draw a diagram of the board representing the blocks in their proper spaces. In all, six measures are obtained. Scoring is based on the time needed to place the blocks on the board with the dominant, the nondominant, and both hands. A fourth measure is the sum of the time taken with the right, left, and both hands. The Memory component of this test is the number of blocks correctly reproduced in the drawing on the board; the Location component is the number of blocks correctly localized in the drawing.

Children's Word-Finding Test (Reitan, 1972; Pajurkova,
Orr, Rourke, & Finlayson, 1976; Rourke & Fisk, 1976)

The test consists of 13 items, each item composed of 5 sentences. Each sentence contains a nonsense word, "Grobnik." The child is required to determine the meaning of the nonsense word through the appreciation of its verbal context. *Score*: total correct. *Task requirement*: verbal problem solving and appreciation of contextual cues. *Stimulus*: spoken words. *Response*: spoken answer.

Underlining Test (Doehring, 1968; Rourke & Orr, 1977;
Rourke & Petrauskas, 1977; Rourke & Gates, 1980)

These tests are intended to assess speed and accuracy of visual discrimination for various kinds of verbal and nonverbal visual stimuli presented singly and in combination. In general, the visual stimulus becomes more verbal and more complex with each succeeding subtest. Subtests 1 and 13 involve the same task in order to permit assessment of practice effect. A final test (14) is administered to control for motor speed. A short practice item is given for each subtest.

Subtest 1: Single Number

The child is required to underline the number 4 each time it appears on a printed page containing a random sequence of 360 single numbers. An example of the number to be identified is printed at the top of the page. A short practice test is given. *Score*: total numbers correctly underlined minus total incorrectly underlined in 30 seconds. *Task requirement*: locating and underlining a particular number interspersed among other numbers. *Stimulus*: random sequences of printed numbers. *Response*: simple underlining response to identify single numbers.

Subtest 2: Single Geometric Forms

The child is required to underline a Greek cross with a pencil each time it appears in random sequence among a series of 235 geometric forms, including squares, stars, circles, and triangles, and so forth. The forms are about ¼″ in height. *Score*: total crosses underlined minus total errors in 30 seconds. *Task requirement*: as in previous subtest, but for identification of a geometric form.

Subtest 3: Single Nonsense Letter

A single nonsense letter is interspersed among 10 structurally similar nonsense letters in a random sequence of 126 letters. *Score*: total correct minus incorrect underlined letters in 60 seconds. *Task requirement*: as in previous subtest, but for identification of a nonsense letter.

Subtest 4: Gestalt Figure

The figure to be identified is a diamond about 8 mm in height containing a square which in turn contains a diamond. This figure is interspersed among similar figures in a random sequence of 168 figures. *Score*: total correct minus incorrect underlined figures in 60 seconds. *Task requirement*: as in previous subtest, but for identification of a complex figure.

Subtest 5: Single Letter

The letter *s* is interspersed among 360 randomized letters. *Score*: number underlined minus number of errors in 30 seconds. *Task requirement*: as in previous subtest, but for a single letter.

Subtest 6: Single Letter in Syllable Context

One hundred sixty-two four-letter nonsense syllables are presented, 47 of which contain the letter *e*. The child is required to underline each syllable containing *e*. *Score*: total correct minus incorrect in 45 seconds. *Task requirement*: as in previous subtest, but for a letter in syllable context.

Subtest 7: Two Letters

The letters *b* and *m* are interspersed among 360 randomized letters. *Score*: number underlined minus number of errors in 45 seconds. *Task requirement*: as in previous subtest, but for two letters.

Subtest 8: Sequence of Geometric Forms

Four geometric forms (triangle, Greek cross, circle, crescent) are presented in various orders for a total of 65 "syllables." The child is required to underline only the groups with the order triangle, cross, crescent, and circle. *Score*: total groups correctly underlined minus errors in 60 seconds. *Task requirement*: same as in previous subtest, but for groups of geometric figures.

Subtest 9: Four-Letter Nonsense Syllable, Unpronounceable

The child is required to underline a four-letter nonsense syllable ("fsbm") interspersed among 146 four-letter nonsense syllables. All syllables are made up of the consonants *f*, *s*, *b*, and *m*, which renders them unpronounceable. *Score*: total correct minus incorrect in 60 seconds. *Task requirement*: same as previous subtest, but for nonsense syllables.

Subtest 10: Four-Letter Nonsense Syllable, Pronounceable

This task is the same as in the previous subtest except that it involves the identification of a pronounceable nonsense syllable ("narp") instead of an unpronounceable nonsense syllable. This syllable is interspersed among other nonsense syllables made up of the letters *n*, *a*, *r*, *p*. *Score*: total correct minus incorrect in 60 seconds. *Task requirement*: same as in previous subtest but for a pronounceable nonsense syllable.

Subtest 11: Four-Letter Word

The word "spot" is interspersed among 146 four-letter syllables made up of the letters *s*, *p*, *o*, *t*. *Score*: total correct minus incorrect in 60 seconds. *Task requirement*: same as in previous subtest, but for a four-letter word.

Subtest 12: Unspaced Four-Letter Word

The word "spot" is interspersed among the letters *s*, *p*, *o*, *t*. *Score*: total correct minus incorrect in 60 seconds. *Task requirement*: same as in previous subtest, but for an unspaced word.

Subtest 13: Single Number

This task is exactly the same as that involved in Subtest 1 except that the number to be underlined is 5 instead of 4.

Subtest 14: Single Rectangle

The child is required to underline a series of identical rectangles, approximately 1 cm $\times$ .5 cm. *Score*: total number underlined in 30 seconds. *Task requirement*: speed of underlining.

YOUNGER CHILDREN'S BATTERY (AGES 5–8)

A. The following tests are the same as those administered to children 9–15 years of age:

- The tactile, auditory, visual, and finger agnosia portions of the Sensory-Perceptual Disturbances Tests
- Target Test
- Sweep Hearing Test
- Auditory Closure Test
- Sentence Memory Test
- Speech-Sounds Perception Test
- Verbal Fluency Test
- Auditory Analysis Test
- Lateral Dominance Examination
- Strength of Grip
- Name-Writing Speed
- Finger- and Foot-Tapping Speed
- Mazes
- Children's Word-Finding Test
- Underlining Test

B. The following tests differ somewhat from those administered to children 9–15 years of age:

Fingertip Symbol-Writing Recognition

The procedure is identical to that described above for Fingertip Number-Writing Perception except that *X*'s and *O*'s are used instead of numbers.

Tactile–Forms Recognition

The child is required to identify familiar forms placed in his/her hands. Four forms are used. Each of these is placed in either hand separately. Then, different pairings of the forms are placed in both hands simultaneously. In all, there are eight possible correct identifications for each hand. *Score*: total incorrect identifications in eight trials for each hand. *Task requirement*: recognition of forms by touch only. *Response*: spoken name of object or pointing to a representation of it.

Halstead–Wepman Aphasia Screening Test (Reitan & Davison, 1974)

Naming (Anomia). Four items. Otherwise, the same.

Writing (Dysgraphia). One item written, one item printed. Otherwise, the same.

Reading (Dyslexia). Three items. Otherwise, the same.

Drawing (Constructional Dyspraxia). Three items. Otherwise, the same.

Arithmetic (Dyscalculia). Four items. Otherwise, the same.

Body Orientation. Four items. The child is required to show or point to his/her nose, tongue, eyebrow, and elbow. *Score*: number of errors.

Right–Left Discrimination. Two items. The child is required to put his/her right hand on his/her nose, and his/her left hand on his/her head. *Score*: number of errors.

Category Test

The Category Test utilizes the same general apparatus and procedure as the Halstead Category Test. However, the test consists of 80 stimulus figures divided into five subtests. The answer panel consists of four answer buttons which are individually identified by red, blue, yellow, and green lights. The principles involved are color, quantity, oddity, and color prominence. As in the Halstead Category Test, the final subtest is of a summary nature and therefore does not have a principle to be discerned.

Graduated Holes Test

The procedure is identical to that described above except that only the four largest holes are used.

Grooved Pegboard Test

The procedure is identical to that described above except that only the first two rows (10 holes) are used.

C. The following tests are used only with children 5–8 years of age:

Color Form Test (Reitan & Davison, 1974)

The Color Form Test uses stimulus material of various colors and shapes. Initially, the child is instructed to follow a sequence of progress from one figure to another by shifting between shape and color as stimulus clues. After a sample, in which careful instruction is given, the test itself is administered. The child moves from the initial figure to one having the same shape even though the color is different, next proceeds to a figure that is different in shape but has the same color, and continues to alternate in this fashion.

Progressive Figures Test (Reitan & Davison, 1974)

This test is presented on an $8\frac{1}{4}'' \times 11''$ sheet of paper on which are printed eight stimulus figures. Each stimulus figure consists of a large outside figure (such as a circle) and a smaller figure of another shape inside (such as a square). The child's task is to use the small inside figure as the clue for progressing to the outside shape of the next stimulus figure. For example, if the child is located at a large circle enclosing a small square, the small square would indicate the next move would be to a large square. If the large square then enclosed a small triangle, the small triangle would serve as a clue for the next move. In this way the child progresses from inside figure to outside figure, moving from one stimulus configuration to the next.

Matching Pictures (Reitan & Davison, 1974)

The test consists of five pages, the first of which is a practice page. The task requires the child to match pictures located at the top of the page with their appropriate pairs shown across the bottom of the page. While the practice items require only matching of identical figures, the test progresses in such a way that a limited degree of generalization is required. For example, on one page a picture of a woman must be used to match the stimulus figure of a man, or a girl to match a boy. On another page a horse matches a cow, a chicken matches a rooster, and so forth. The test is so organized that it requires the child to respond in terms of equivalent categories in order to perform the test correctly.

Matching Figures and Matching V's (Reitan & Davison, 1974)

The child is asked to match figures printed on little blocks with the same figures printed on a single card. These figures become progressively more complex along the card. The little blocks are presented to each subject in a standardized manner. The score is the time in seconds required to complete the task, and the number of errors.

Drawing of Star and Concentric Squares (Reitan & Davison, 1974)

The child is required to copy the figure presented to him/her. The examiner points out specifically how the figure is made up. The score is the time in seconds required to complete each drawing, and the number of errors in each drawing.

References

Ackerman, D., & Howes, C. (1986). Sociometric status and after-school activity of children with learning disabilities. *Journal of Learning Disabilities, 19*, 416–419.

Anderson, S., & Messick, S. (1974). Social competency in young children. *Developmental Psychology, 10*, 282–293.

Applebee, A. N. (1971). Research in reading retardation: Two critical problems. *Journal of Child Psychology and Psychiatry, 12*, 91–113.

Bachara, G. (1976). Empathy in learning disabled children. *Perceptual and Motor Skills, 43*, 541–542.

Bakker, D. J. (1979). Perceptual asymmetries and reading proficiency. In M. Bortner (Ed.), *Cognitive growth and development: Essays in memory of Herbert G. Birch* (pp. 134–152). New York: Brunner/Mazel.

Barnes, R. (1986). The recurrent self-harm patient. *Suicide and Life-Threatening Behavior, 16*, 399–408.

Baron, I. S. (1987). The childhood presentation of social-emotional learning disabilities: On the continuum of Asperger's syndrome [Abstract]. *Journal of Clinical and Experimental Neuropsychology, 9*, 30.

Benson, D. F., & Geschwind, N. (1970). Developmental Gerstmann syndrome. *Neurology, 20*, 293–298.

Benton, A. L. (1965). *Sentence Memory Test.* Iowa City, IA: Author.

Benton, A. L. (1975). Developmental dyslexia: Neurological aspects. In W. J. Friedlander (Ed.), *Advances in neurology* (Vol. 7, pp. 1–41). New York: Raven Press.

Black, F. W. (1974). Self-concept as related to achievement and age in learning disabled children. *Child Development, 45*, 1137–1140.

Brandys, C., Rourke, B. P., & Shore, D. L. (1989). Memory functions in reading- and arithmetic-disabled children. Manuscript in preparation.

Breen, M. J., & Barkley, R. A. (1984). Psychological adjustment in learning-disabled, hyperactive, and hyperactive/learning-disabled children as measured by the Personality Inventory for Children. *Journal of Clinical Child Psychology, 13*, 232–236.

Bruininks, V. L. (1978). Peer status and personality characteristics of learning disabled and nondisabled students. *Journal of Learning Disabilities, 11*, 29–34.

Bryan, T. H. (1974a). An observational analysis of classroom behaviors of children with learning disabilities. *Journal of Learning Disabilities, 7*, 26–34.

Bryan, T. H. (1974b). Peer popularity of learning-disabled children. *Journal of Learning Disabilities, 7*, 621–625.

Bryan, T. H. (1976). Peer popularity of learning-disabled children: A replication. *Journal of Learning Disabilities, 9*, 307–311.

Bryan, T. H. (1977). Learning disabled children's comprehension of nonverbal communication. *Journal of Learning Disabilities, 10*, 501–506.

Bryan, T. H. (1982, April). *Social cognitive understanding and language.* Paper presented at the meeting of the Ontario Association for Children with Learning Disabilities, Toronto.

Bryan, T. H., Donohue, M., & Pearl, R. (1981). Learning disabled children's communicative competence on referential communication tasks. *Journal of Pediatric Psychology, 6,* 383–393.

Bryan, T. H., & McGrady, H. J. (1972). Use of a teacher rating scale. *Journal of Learning Disabilities, 5,* 199–206.

Bryan, T. H., & Wheeler, R. (1972). Perception of learning disabled children: The eye of the observer. *Journal of Learning Disabilities, 5,* 484–488.

Campbell, D. M. (1972). Interaction patterns in families with learning problem children. *Dissertation Abstracts International, 33,* 1783B. (University Microfilms No. 72-25, 252)

Casey, J., & Rourke, B. P. (1989). Syndrome of nonverbal learning disabilities: Age differences in neuropsychological skills and abilities. Manuscript in preparation.

Casey, P. (1977). Minimal brain dysfunction in suicide adolescents [Letter to editor]. *Journal of Pediatrics, 91,* 1029–1030.

Cicchetti, D. V., Sparrow, S. S., & Rourke, B. P. (in press). Adaptive behavior profiles of psychologically disturbed and developmentally disabled persons. In R. P. Barrett & J. L. Matson (Eds.), *Research in developmental disabilities annual series.* Greenwich, CT: JAI Press.

Connolly, C. (1969). The psychosocial adjustment of children with dyslexia. *Exceptional Children, 36,* 126–127.

Connolly, C. (1971). Social and emotional factors in learning disabilities. In H. R. Myklebust (Ed.), *Progress in learning disabilities* (Vol. 2, pp. 151–178). New York: Grune & Stratton.

Copeland, D. R., Fletcher, J. M., Pfefferbaum-Levine, B., Jaffe, M., Ried, H., & Maor, M. (1985). Neuropsychological sequelae of childhood cancer in long-term survivors. *Pediatrics, 75,* 745–753.

Corballis, M. C., & Morgan, M. J. (1978). On the biological basis of human laterality: I. Evidence for a maturational left–right gradient. *Behavioral and Brain Sciences, 2,* 261–336.

Cowen, E. L., Pederson, A., Babigian, H., Izzo, L. D., & Trost, M. A. (1973). Long-term follow-up of early detected vulnerable children. *Journal of Consulting and Clinical Psychology, 41,* 438–446.

Czudner, G., & Rourke, B. P. (1972). Age differences in visual reaction time in "brain-damaged" and normal children under regular and irregular preparatory interval conditions. *Journal of Experimental Child Psychology, 13,* 516–526.

Del Dotto, J. E., Rourke, B. P., McFadden, G. T., & Fisk, J. L. (1987). Developmental analysis of arithmetic-disabled children: Impact on personality adjustment and patterns of adaptive functioning [Abstract]. *Journal of Clinical and Experimental Neuropsychology, 9,* 44.

Dennis, M. (1977). Cerebral dominance in three forms of early brain disorder. In M. E. Blaw, I. Rapin, & M. Kinsbourne (Eds.), *Topics in child neurology* (pp. 189–212). New York: Spectrum.

Dennis, M. (1981). Language in a congenitally acallosal brain. *Brain and Language, 12,* 33–53.

Dennis, M., Hendrick, E. B., Hoffman, H. J., & Humphreys, R. P. (1987). Language of hydrocephalic children and adolescents. *Journal of Clinical and Experimental Neuropsychology, 9,* 593–621.

Doehring, D. G. (1968). *Patterns of impairment in specific reading disability.* Bloomington: Indiana University Press.

Doehring, D. G. (1978). The tangled web of behavioral research on developmental dyslexia. In A. L. Benton & D. Pearl (Eds.), *Dyslexia: An appraisal of current knowledge* (pp. 125–135). New York: Oxford University Press.

Doehring, D. G., & Hoshko, I. M. (1977). Classification of reading problems by the *Q*-technique of factor analysis. *Cortex, 13*, 281–294.

Doehring, D. G., Hoshko, I. M., & Bryans, B. N. (1979). Statistical classification of children with reading problems. *Journal of Clinical Neuropsychology, 1*, 5–16.

Doll, E. A. (1953). *Vineland Social Maturity Scale.* Minneapolis: Educational Test Bureau.

Dunn, L. M. (1965). *Expanded manual for the Peabody Picture Vocabulary Test.* Minneapolis: American Guidance Services.

Ewing-Cobbs, L., Fletcher, J. M., & Levin, H. S. (1985). Neuropsychological sequelae following pediatric head injury. In M. Ylvisaker (Ed.), *Closed head injury rehabilitation: Children and adolescents* (pp. 71–89). San Diego: College Hill.

Fein, D., Pennington, B., Markowitz, P., Braverman, M., & Waterhouse, L. (1986). Toward a neuropsychological model of infantile autism: Are the social deficits primary? *Journal of the American Academy of Child Psychiatry, 25*, 198–212.

Fisk, J. L., & Rourke, B. P. (1979). Identification of subtypes of learning-disabled children at three age levels: A neuropsychological, multivariate approach. *Journal of Clinical Neuropsychology, 1*, 289–310.

Fletcher, J. M. (1985). External validation of learning disability typologies. In B. P. Rourke (Ed.), *Neuropsychology of learning disabilities: Essentials of subtype analysis* (pp. 187–211). New York: Guilford Press.

Fletcher, J. M., & Copeland, D. R. (1988). Neurobehavioral effects of central nervous system prophylactic treatment of cancer in children. *Journal of Clinical and Experimental Neuropsychology, 10*, 495–537.

Fletcher, J. M., & Levin, H. S. (1988). Neurobehavioral effects of brain injury in children. In D. K. Routh (Ed.), *Handbook of pediatric psychology* (pp. 258–295). New York: Guilford Press.

Fletcher, J. M., & Satz, P. (1980). Developmental changes in the neuropsychological correlates of reading achievement: A six-year longitudinal follow-up. *Journal of Clinical Neuropsychology, 2*, 23–37.

Fletcher, J. M., & Taylor, H. G. (1984). Neuropsychological approaches to children: Towards a developmental neuropsychology. *Journal of Clinical Neuropsychology, 6*, 39–56.

Freud, S. (1974). A case of homosexuality in a woman. In J. Strachey (Ed. & Trans.), *The standard edition of the complete psychological works of Sigmund Freud* (Vol. 18, pp. 146–262). London: Hogarth Press. (Original work published 1920)

Fuerst, D., Fisk, J. L., & Rourke, B. P. (1989a). Psychosocial functioning of learning-disabled children: Replicability of statistically derived subtypes. *Journal of Consulting and Clinical Psychology, 57.*

Fuerst, D., Fisk, J. L., & Rourke, B. P. (1989b). Psychosocial functioning of learning-disabled children: Relationships between personality subtypes and WISC Verbal IQ–Performance IQ discrepancies. *Journal of Consulting and Clinical Psychology* (under review).

Galaburda, A. M., LeMay, M., Kemper, T. L., & Geschwind, N. (1978). Right–left asymmetries in the brain. *Science, 199*, 852–856.

Goldberg, E., & Costa, L. D. (1981). Hemisphere differences in the acquisition and use of descriptive systems. *Brain and Language, 14*, 144–173.

Goldman, M., & Barclay, A. (1974). Influence of maternal attitudes on children with reading disabilities. *Perceptual and Motor Skills, 38*, 303–307.

Grunebaum, M. G., Hurwitz, I., Prentice, M. M., & Sperry, B. M. (1962). Fathers of sons with primary neurotic learning inhibitions. *American Journal of Orthopsychiatry*, *32*, 462–472.

Gur, R. C., Pack, I. K. Hungerbuhler, J. P., Reivich, M., Obrist, W. D., Amarnet, W. S., & Sackeim, H. A. (1980). Differences in the distribution of gray and white matter in human cerebral hemispheres. *Science, 207*, 1226–1228.

Halechko, A. D. (1977). Self-esteem and perception of parental behavior in children with learning disabilities. *Dissertation Abstracts International, 38*, 359B. (University Microfilms No. 77-15, 246)

Halstead, W. C. (1947). *Brain and intelligence.* Chicago: University of Chicago Press.

Harris, A. T. (1947). *Harris Tests of Lateral Dominance. Manual of directions for administration and interpretation.* New York: Psychological Corp.

Hebb, D. O. (1949). *Organization of behavior.* New York: John Wiley.

Heilman, K. M., & Van Den Abell, T. (1979). Right hemispheric dominance for mediating cerebral activation. *Neuropsychologia, 17*, 315–321.

Heilman, K. M., & Van Den Abell, T. (1980). Right hemispheric dominance for attention: The mechanism underlying hemispheric asymmetries of inattention (neglect). *Neurology, 30*, 317–330.

Hendin, H. (1985). Suicide among the young: Psychodynamics and demography. In M. Peck, N. L. Farberow, & R. E. Litman (Eds.), *Youth suicide* (pp. 19–38). New York: Springer.

Holland, C. J. (1983). *Directive Parental Counseling: The counselor's guide.* Bloomfield Hills, MI: Midwest Professional Publishing.

Hutchinson, E. D. (1949a). The nature of insight. In P. Mullahy (Ed.), *A study of interpersonal relations: New contributions to psychiatry* (421–445). New York: Grove Press.

Hutchinson, E. D. (1949b). The period of frustration in creative endeavor. In P. Mullahy (Ed.), *A study of interpersonal relations: New contributions to psychiatry* (pp. 404–420). New York: Grove Press.

Jastak, J. F., & Jastak, S. R. (1965). *The Wide Range Achievement Test.* Wilmington, DE: Guidance Associates.

Johnson, D. J., & Myklebust, H. R. (1967). *Learning disabilities.* New York: Grune & Stratton.

Kass, C. E. (1964). Auditory Closure Test. In J. J. Olson & J. L. Olson (Eds.), *Validity studies on the Illinois Test of Psycholinguistic Abilities.* Madison, WI: Photo.

Kenny, T. J., Rohn, R., Sarles, R. M., Reynolds, F. J. & Heald, F. P. (1979). Visual–motor problems of adolescents who attempt suicide. *Perceptual and Motor Skills, 48*, 599–602.

Keogh, B. K., Tchir, C., & Windeguth-Behn, A. (1974). Teachers' perceptions of educationally high risk children. *Journal of Learning Disabilities, 7*, 43–50.

Kertesz, A., & Dobrowolski, S. (1981). Right-hemisphere deficits, lesion size and location. *Journal of Clinical Neuropsychiatry, 3*, 283–299.

Kinsbourne, M., & Warrington, E. K. (1963). The developmental Gerstmann syndrome. *Archives of Neurology, 8*, 490–501.

Kirk, S. A., & McCarthy, J. J. (1961). The Illinois Test of Psycholinguistic Abilities: An approach to differential diagnosis. *American Journal of Mental Deficiency, 66*, 399–412.

Klove, H. (1963). Clinical neuropsychology. In F. M. Forster (Ed.), *The medical clinics of North America* (pp. 1647–1658). New York: Saunders.

Knights, R. M., & Moule, A. D. (1967). Normative and reliability data on finger and foot tapping in children. *Perceptual and Motor Skills, 25*, 717–720.

Knights, R. M., & Moule, A. D. (1968). Normative data on the Motor Steadiness Battery for Children. *Perceptual and Motor Skills, 26*, 643–650.

Knights, R. M., & Norwood, J. A. (1980). Revised smoothed normative data on the neuropsychological test battery for children. Carleton University, Department of Psychology, Ottawa, Ontario.

Kronick, D. (1980). An overview of research relating to the etiology of interactional deficits in the learning disabled. In R. M. Knights & D. J. Bakker (Eds.), *Treatment of hyperactive and learning disordered children* (pp. 395–407). Baltimore: University Park Press.

La Greca, A. M. (1981). Social behavior and social perception in learning-disabled children: A review with implications for social skills training. *Journal of Pediatric Psychology, 6*, 395–416.

Lashley, K. S. (1938). Factors limiting recovery after central nervous system lesions. *Journal of Nervous and Mental Diseases, 88*, 733–755.

Leenaars, A. A. (1988). *Suicide notes.* New York: Human Sciences Press.

Leenaars, A. A. (in press). Suicide in the school-age child. In A. Leenaars & D. Lester (Eds.), *Suicide across the life-span.* New York: Human Sciences Press.

Leenaars, A. A., Balance, W. D. G., Wenckstern, S., & Rudzinski, D. (1985). An empirical investigation of Shneidman's formulations regarding suicide. *Suicide and Life-Threatening Behavior, 15*, 184–195.

LeMay, M. (1976). Morphological cerebral asymmetries of modern man, fossil man, and nonhuman primate. In S. R. Harnad, H. D. Steklis, & J. Lancaster (Eds.), *Origins and evolution of language and speech. Annals of the New York Academy of Sciences, 280*, 349–366.

LeMay, M., & Culebras, A. (1972). Human brain: Morphologic differences in the hemispheres demonstrable by carotid arteriography. *New England Journal of Medicine, 287*, 168–170.

Lorin, R. P., Cowen, E. L., & Caldwell, R. A. (1974). Problem types of children referred to a school-based mental health program: Identification and outcome. *Journal of Consulting and Clinical Psychology, 47*, 491–496.

Luria, A. R. (1966). *Higher cortical functions in man.* New York: Basic Books.

Lyon, R. (1985). Educational validation studies of learning disability subtypes. In B. P. Rourke (Ed.), *Learning disabilities in children: Advances in subtype analysis* (pp. 228–253). New York: Guilford Press.

MacDonald, G. W., & Roy, D. L. (1988). Williams syndrome: A neuropsychological profile. *Journal of Clinical and Experimental Neuropsychology, 10*, 125–131.

Maris, R. (1985). The adolescent suicide problem. *Suicide and Life-Threatening Behavior, 15*, 91–109.

Maris, R. (Ed.). (1986). *Biology of suicide.* New York: Guilford Press.

Mattis, S., French, J. H., & Rapin, I. (1975). Dyslexia in children and young adults: Three independent neuropsychological syndromes. *Developmental Medicine and Child Neurology, 17*, 150–163.

McCarthy, J. M., & Paraskevopoulos, J. (1969). Behavior patterns of learning disabled, emotionally disturbed, and average children. *Exceptional Children, 36*, 69–74.

McConaughty, S. H., & Ritter, D. R. (1986). Social competence and behavioral problems of learning disabled boys aged 6–11. *Journal of Learning Disabilities, 19*, 39–45.

McKinney, J. D., Short, E. J., & Feagans, L. (1985). Academic consequences of perceptual-linguistic subtypes of learning disabled children. *Learning Disabilities Research, 1*, 6–17.

McKinney, J. D., & Speece, D. L. (1986). Academic consequences and longitudinal stability of behavioral subtypes of learning disabled children. *Journal of Educational Psychology, 78*, 365–372.

McNutt, G. L. (1978). The identification of learning disabled adolescents. *Dissertation Abstracts International, 38*, 4097A. (University Microfilms No. 77-29, 067)

Menninger, K. A. (1938). *Man against himself.* New York: Harcourt, Brace.

Miles, W. R. (1929). *The A-B-C Vision Test.* New York: Psychological Corp.

Miller, D. R., & Westman, J. C. (1964). Reading disability as a condition of family stability. *Family Process, 3,* 66–76.

Morris, R., Blashfield, R., & Satz, P. (1981). Neuropsychology and cluster analysis: Potentials and problems. *Journal of Clinical Neuropsychology, 3,* 79–99.

Morris, R., Blashfield, R., & Satz, P. (1986). Developmental classification of reading-disabled children. *Journal of Clinical and Experimental Neuropsychology, 8,* 371–392.

Morris, R., & Fletcher, J. M. (1988). Classification in neuropsychology: A Theoretical framework and research paradigm. *Journal of Clinical and Experimental Neuropsychology, 10,* 640–658.

Murray, H. (1967). Dead to the world: The passions of Herman Melville. In E. Shneidman (Ed.), *Essays in self-destruction* (pp. 7–29). New York: Science House.

Myklebust, H. R. (1975). Nonverbal learning disabilities: Assessment and intervention. In H. R. Myklebust (Ed.), *Progress in learning disabilities* (Vol. 3, pp. 85–121). New York: Grune & Stratton.

Nakamura, C. Y., & Finck, D. N. (1980). Relative effectiveness of socially oriented and task-oriented children and predictability of their behaviors. *Monographs of the Society for Research in Child Development, 45* (No. 185).

Natchez, G. (Ed.). (1968). *Children with reading problems.* New York: Basic Books.

Owen, F. W., Adams, P. A., Forrest, T., Stolz, L. M., & Fisher, S. (1971). Learning disorders in children: Sibling studies. *Monographs of the Society for Research in Child Development, 36*(No. 144).

Ozols, E. J., & Rourke, B. P. (1985). Dimensions of social sensitivity in two types of learning-disabled children. In B. P. Rourke (Ed.), *Neuropsychology of learning disabilities: Essentials of subtype analysis* (pp. 281–301). New York: Guilford Press.

Ozols, E. J., & Rourke, B. P. (1988). Characteristics of young learning-disabled children classified according to patterns of academic achievement: Auditory-perceptual and visual-perceptual abilities. *Journal of Clinical Child Psychology, 17,* 44–52.

Ozols, E. J., & Rourke, B. P. (in press). Classification of young learning-disabled children according to patterns of academic achievement. In B. P. Rourke (Ed.), *Neuropsychological validation of learning disability subtypes.* New York: Guilford Press.

Pajurkova, E., Orr, R. R., Rourke, B. P., & Finlayson, M. A. J. (1976). Children's Word-Finding Test: A verbal problem-solving task. *Perceptual and Motor Skills, 42,* 851–858.

Peck, B. B., & Stackhouse, T. (1973). Reading problems and family dynamics. *Journal of Learning Disabilities, 6,* 506–511.

Peck, M. (1985). Crisis intervention treatment with chronically and acutely suicidal adolescents. In M. Peck, N. L. Farberow, & R. E. Litman (Eds.), *Youth suicide* (pp. 112–122). New York: Springer.

Peter, B. M., & Spreen, O. (1979). Behavior rating and personal adjustment scales of neurologically and learning handicapped children during adolescence and early adulthood: Results of a follow-up study. *Journal of Clinical Neuropsychology, 1,* 75–91.

Petrauskas, R. J., & Rourke, B. P. (1979). Identification of subtypes of retarded readers: A neuropsychological, multivariate approach. *Journal of Clinical Neuropsychology, 1,* 17–37.

Piaget, J. (1954). *The construction of reality in the child.* New York: Basic Books.

Porter, J. E., & Rourke, B. P. (1985). Socioemotional functioning of learning-disabled children: A subtypal analysis of personality patterns. In B. P. Rourke (Ed.),

Neuropsychology of learning disabilities: Essentials of subtype analysis (pp. 257–279). New York: Guilford Press.

Quay, H. C. (1972). Patterns of aggression, withdrawal, and immaturity. In H. C. Quay & J. S. Werry (Eds.), *Psychopathological disorders of childhood* (pp. 1–29). New York: John Wiley.

Reitan, R. M. (1966). A research program on the psychological effects of brain lesions in human beings. In N. R. Ellis (Ed.), *International review of research in mental retardation* (pp. 153–218). New York: Academic Press.

Reitan, R. M. (1972). Verbal problem-solving as related to brain damage. *Perceptual and Motor Skills, 34*, 515–524.

Reitan, R. M. (1974a). Methodological problems in clinical neuropsychology. In R. M. Reitan & L. A. Davison (Eds.), *Clinical neuropsychology: Current status and applications* (pp. 19–46). Washington, DC: V. H. Winston.

Reitan, R. M., & Davison, L. A. (Eds.). (1974). *Clinical neuropsychology: Current status and applications*. Washington, DC: V. H. Winston.

Ribner, S. (1978). The effects of special class placement on the self-concept of exceptional children. *Journal of Learning Disabilities, 11*, 319–323.

Richey, D. D., & McKinney, J. D. (1978). Classroom behavioral subtypes of learning disabled boys. *Journal of Learning Disabilities, 11*, 297–302.

Robins, L. N., West, P. A., & Murphy, G. E. (1977). The high rate of suicide in older white men: A study testing the hypothesis. *Social Psychiatry, 12*, 1–20.

Rohn, R., Sarles, R. M., Kenny, R. J., Reynolds, J. R., & Heald, F. P. (1977). Adolescents who attempt suicide. *Journal of Pediatrics, 90*, 636–638.

Rosner, J., & Simon, D. P. (1970). *Auditory Analysis Test: An initial report*. Pittsburgh: Author, University of Pittsburgh, Learning Research and Development Center.

Rourke, B. P. (1975). Brain–behavior relationships in children with learning disabilities: A research program. *American Psychologist, 30*, 911–920.

Rourke, B. P. (1976a). Issues in the neuropsychological assessment of children with learning disabilities. *Canadian Psychological Review, 17*, 89–102.

Rourke, B. P. (1976b). Reading retardation in children: Developmental lag or deficit? In R. M. Knights & D. J. Bakker (Eds.), *Neuropsychology of learning disorders: Theoretical approaches* (pp. 125–137). Baltimore: University Park Press.

Rourke, B. P. (1978a). Neuropsychological research in reading retardation: A review. In A. L. Benton & D. Pearl (Eds.), *Dyslexia: An appraisal of current knowledge* (pp. 141–171). New York: Oxford University Press.

Rourke, B. P. (1978b). Reading, spelling, arithmetic disabilities: A neuropsychological perspective. In H. R. Myklebust (Ed.), *Progress in learning disabilities* (Vol. 4, pp. 97–120). New York: Grune & Stratton.

Rourke, B. P. (1980). Conference overview. In R. M. Knights & D. J. Bakker (Eds.), *Treatment of hyperactive and learning disordered children: Current research* (pp. xiii–xvi). Baltimore: University Park Press.

Rourke, B. P. (1981). Neuropsychological assessment of children with learning disabilities. In S. B. Filskov & T. J. Boll (Eds.), *Handbook of clinical neuropsychology* (pp. 453–478). New York: Wiley-Interscience.

Rourke, B. P. (1982). Central processing deficiencies in children: Toward a developmental neuropsychological model. *Journal of Clinical Neuropsychology, 4*, 1–18.

Rourke, B. P. (1983a). Outstanding issues in research in learning disabilities. In M. Rutter (Ed.), *Developmental neuropsychiatry* (pp. 564–574). New York: Guilford Press.

Rourke, B. P. (1983b). Reading and spelling disabilities: A developmental neuropsychological perspective. In U. Kirk (Ed.), *Neuropsychology of language, reading, and spelling* (pp. 209–234). New York: Academic Press.

Rourke, B. P. (Ed.). (1985). *Neuropsychology of learning disabilities: Essentials of subtype analysis.* New York: Guilford Press.

Rourke, B. P. (1987). Syndrome of nonverbal learning disabilities: The final common pathway of white-matter disease/dysfunction? *The Clinical Neuropsychologist, 1,* 209–234.

Rourke, B. P. (1988a). Socioemotional disturbances of learning-disabled children. *Journal of Consulting and Clinical Psychology, 56,* 801–810.

Rourke, B. P. (1988b). Syndrome of nonverbal learning disabilities: Developmental manifestations in neurological disease, disorder, and dysfunction. *The Clinical Neuropsychologist, 2,* 293–330.

Rourke, B. P., & Adams, K. M. (1984). Quantitative approaches to the neuropsychological assessment of children. In R. M. Tarter & G. Goldstein (Eds.), *Advances in clinical neuropsychology* (Vol. 2, pp. 79–108). New York: Plenum.

Rourke, B. P., Bakker, D. J., Fisk, J. L., & Strang, J. D. (1983). *Child neuropsychology: An introduction to theory, research, and clinical practice.* New York: Guilford Press.

Rourke, B. P., & Casey, J. (1989). Syndrome of nonverbal learning disabilities: Age difference in personality/behavioral functioning. Manuscript in preparation.

Rourke, B. P., Czudner, G. (1972). Age differences in auditory reaction time of "brain-damaged" and normal children under regular and irregular preparatory interval conditions. *Journal of Experimental Child Psychology, 14,* 372–378.

Rourke, B. P., Dietrich, D. M., & Young, G. C. (1973). Significance of WISC Verbal-Performance discrepancies for younger children with learning disabilities. *Perceptual and Motor Skills, 36,* 275–282.

Rourke, B. P., & Finlayson, M. A. J. (1978). Neuropsychological significance of variations in patterns of academic performance: Verbal and visual-spatial abilities. *Journal of Abnormal Child Psychology, 6,* 121–133.

Rourke, B. P., & Fisk, J. L. (1976). *Children's Word-Finding Test (Revised).* Windsor, Ontario: Author, University of Windsor, Department of Psychology.

Rourke, B. P., & Fisk, J. L. (1981). Socio-emotional disturbances of learning disabled children: The role of central processing deficits. *Bulletin of the Orton Society, 31,* 77–88.

Rourke, B. P., & Fisk, J. L. (1988). Subtypes of learning-disabled children: Implications for a neurodevelopmental model of differential hemispheric processing. In D. L. Molfese & S. J. Segalowitz (Eds.), *Brain lateralization in children: Developmental implications* (pp. 547–565). New York: Guilford Press.

Rourke, B. P., Fisk, J. L., & Strang, J. D. (1986). *Neuropsychological assessment of children: A treatment-oriented approach.* New York: Guilford Press.

Rourke, B. P., & Gates, R. D. (1980). *Underlining Test: Preliminary norms.* Windsor, Ontario: Author, University of Windsor, Department of Psychology.

Rourke, B. P., & Gates, R. D. (1981). Neuropsychological research and school psychology. In G. W. Hynd & J. E. Obrzut (Eds.), *Neuropsychological assessment and the school-aged child: Issues and procedures* (pp. 3–25). New York: Grune & Stratton.

Rourke, B. P., & Orr, R. R. (1977). Predictions of the reading and spelling performances of normal and retarded readers: A four-year follow-up. *Journal of Abnormal Child Psychology, 5,* 9–20.

Rourke, B. P., & Petrauskas, R. J. (1977). *Underlining Test (Revised).* Windsor, Ontario: Author, University of Windsor, Department of Psychology.

Rourke, B. P., Pohlman, C. L., Fuerst, D. R., Porter, J. E., & Fisk, J. L. (1985). Personality subtypes of learning-disabled children: Two validation studies [Abstract]. *Journal of Clinical and Experimental Neuropsychology, 7,* 157.

Rourke, B. P., & Russell, D. L. (1989). Phonetic accuracy of misspellings: Concurrent and predictive validity in normal and disabled readers and spellers. Manuscript in preparation.

Rourke, B. P., & Strang, J. D. (1978). Neuropsychological significance of variations in patterns of academic performance: Motor, psychomotor, and tactile-perceptual abilities. *Journal of Pediatric Psychology, 3*, 62–66.

Rourke, B. P., & Strang, J. D. (1983). Subtypes of reading and arithmetical disabilities: A neuropsychological analysis. In M. Rutter (Ed.), *Developmental neuropsychiatry* (pp. 473–488). New York: Guilford Press.

Rourke, B. P., & Telegdy, G. A. (1971). Lateralizing significance of WISC Verbal–Performance discrepancies for older children with learning disabilities. *Perceptual and Motor Skills, 33*, 875–883.

Rourke, B. P., Yanni, D. W., MacDonald, G. W., & Young, G. C. (1973). Neuropsychological significance of lateralized deficits on the Grooved Pegboard Test for older children with learning disabilities. *Journal of Consulting and Clinical Psychology, 41*, 128–134.

Rourke, B. P., Young, G. C., & Flewelling, R. W. (1971). The relationships between WISC Verbal Performance discrepancies and selected verbal, auditory-perceptual, and problem-solving abilities in children with learning disabilities. *Journal of Clinical Psychology, 27*, 475–479.

Rourke, B. P., Young, G. C., & Leenaars, A. A. (1989). A childhood learning disability that predisposes those afflicted to adolescent and adult depression and suicide risk. *Journal of Learning Disabilities, 22*.

Rourke, B. P., Young, G. C., Strang, J. D., & Russell, D. L. (1986). Adult outcomes of central processing deficiencies in childhood. In I. Grant & K. M. Adams (Eds.), *Neuropsychological assessment in neuropsychiatric disorders: Clinical methods and empirical findings* (pp. 244–267). New York: Oxford University Press.

Routh, D. K., & Mesibov, G. B. (1980). Psychological and environmental intervention. In H. F. Rie & E. D. Rie (Eds.), *Handbook of minimal brain dysfunctions* (pp. 618–644). New York: John Wiley.

Russell, D. L., & Rourke, B. P. (1989). Phonetic accuracy of misspellings: Neuropsychological significance in normal and disabled readers and spellers. *Brain and Language* (under review).

Russell, D. L., Rourke, B. P., & Knights, R. M. (1989). Neuropsychological characteristics of normal and disabled readers and spellers: A profile analytic approach. Manuscript in preparation.

Rutter, M. (1982). Developmental neuropsychiatry: Concept, issues, and prospects. *Journal of Clinical Neuropsychology, 4*, 91–115.

Schaefer, E. S., Edgerton, M., & Aronson, M. (1977). *Classroom Behavior Inventory.* Chapel Hill, NC: The Frank Porter Graham Child Development Center.

Seigler, H. G., & Gynther, M. D. (1960). Reading ability of children and family harmony. *Journal of Developmental Reading, 4*, 17–24.

Shneidman, E. (1985). *Definition of suicide.* New York: John Wiley.

Siegel, E. (1974). *The exceptional child grows up.* New York: E. P. Dutton.

Silverman, R. G. (1978). An investigation of self concept in urban, suburban and rural students with learning disabilities. *Dissertation Abstracts International, 38*, 5398A. (University Microfilms No. 78-01, 877)

Simpson, M. A. (1975). Unrecognized drug-induced dystonias. *Activitas Nervosa Superia, 17*, 79–80.

Sipperstein, G. N., Bopp, M. A., & Bak, J. J. (1978). Social status of learning disabled children. *Journal of Learning Disabilities, 11*, 98–102.

Smith, W. L. (1982). The thirteenth nerve: "A right to love and a right to die." *Clinical Neuropsychology, 4*, 175–176.

Sparrow, S. S., Balla, D. A., & Cicchetti, D. B. (1984). *The Vineland Adaptive Behavior Scales; A revision of the Vineland Social Maturity Scale by Edgar A. Doll.* Circle Pines, MN: American Guidance Services.

Speece, D. L., McKinney, J. D., & Appelbaum, M. I. (1985). Classification and validation of behavioral subtypes of learning-disabled children. *Journal of Educational Psychology, 77*, 67–77.

Stag, G. A. (1972). Comparative behavioral ratings of parents with severely mentally retarded, specific learning disability and normal children. *Journal of Learning Disabilities, 5*, 631–635.

Stevens, D. E., & Moffitt, T. E. (1988). Neuropsychological profile of an Asperger's syndrome case with exceptional calculating ability. *The Clinical Neuropsychologist, 2*, 228–238.

Strang, J. D. (1981). *Personality dimensions of learning-disabled children: Age and subtype differences.* Unpublished doctoral dissertation, University of Windsor, Windsor, Ontario.

Strang, J. D., & Rourke, B. P. (1983). Concept-formation/non-verbal reasoning abilities of children who exhibit specific academic problems with arithmetic. *Journal of Clinical Child Psychology, 12*, 33–39.

Strang, J. D., & Rourke, B. P. (1985a). Adaptive behavior of children with specific arithmetic disabilities and associated neuropsychological abilities and deficits. In B. P. Rourke (Ed.), *Neuropsychology of learning disabilities: Essentials of subtype analysis* (pp. 302–328). New York: Guilford Press.

Strang, J. D., & Rourke, B. P. (1985b). Arithmetic disability subtypes: The neuropsychological significance of specific arithmetic impairment in childhood. In B. P. Rourke (Ed.), *Neuropsychology of learning disabilities: Essentials of subtype analysis* (pp. 167–183). New York: Guilford Press.

Sweeney, J. E., & Rourke, B. P. (1978). Neuropsychological significance of phonetically accurate and phonetically inaccurate spelling errors in younger and older retarded spellers. *Brain and Language, 6*, 212–225.

Sweeney, J. E., & Rourke, B. P. (1985). Spelling disability subtypes. In B. P. Rourke (Ed.), *Neuropsychology of learning disabilities: Essentials of subtype analysis* (pp. 147–166). New York: Guilford Press.

Taylor, H. G. (1983). MBD: Meanings and misconceptions. *Journal of Clinical Neuropsychology, 5*, 271–288.

Taylor, H. G. (1984). Early brain injury and cognitive development. In C. R. Almli & S. Finger (Eds.), *Early brain damage: Research orientations and clinical observations* (Vol. 1, pp. 323–345). New York: Academic Press.

Taylor, H. G. (1987). Childhood sequelae of early neurological disorders: A contemporary perspective. *Developmental Neuropsychology, 3*, 153–164.

Taylor, H. G., Albo, V. C., Phebus, C. K., Sachs, B. R., & Bierl, P. G. (1987). Postirradiation treatment outcomes for children with acute lymphocytic leukemia: Clarification of risks. *Journal of Pediatric Psychology, 12*, 395–411.

Taylor, H. G., & Fletcher, J. M. (1983). Biological foundations of specific developmental disorders: Methods, findings, and future directions. *Journal of Clinical Child Psychology, 12*, 46–65.

Tranel, D., Hall, L. E., Olson, S., & Tranel, N. N. (1987). Evidence for a right-hemisphere developmental learning disability. *Developmental Neuropsychology, 3*, 113–127.

Van Zomeren, A. H. (1981). *Reaction time and attention after closed head injury.* Lisse, The Netherlands: Swetz and Zeitlinger.

Voeller, K. K. S. (1986). Right-hemisphere deficit syndrome in children. *American Journal of Psychiatry, 143,* 1004–1009.

Wada, J. A., Clarke, R., & Hamm, A. (1975). Cerebral hemispheric asymmetry in humans. *Archives of Neurology, 32,* 239–246.

Wechsler, D. (1949). *Wechsler Intelligence Scale for Children.* New York: Psychological Corp.

Weintraub, S., & Mesulam, M. M. (1983). Developmental learning disabilities of the right hemisphere: Emotional, interpersonal, and cognitive components. *Archives of Neurology, 40,* 463–468.

Wetter, J. (1972). Parental attitudes toward learning disability. *Exceptional Children, 38,* 490–491.

Wiener, J. (1980). A theoretical model of the acquisition of peer relations of learning disabled children. *Journal of Learning Disabilities, 13,* 42–47.

Wiig, E. H., & Harris, S. P. (1974). Perception and interpretation of nonverbally expressed emotions by adolescents with learning disabilities. *Perceptual and Motor Skills, 38,* 239–245.

Wing, L. (1981). Asperger's syndrome: A clinical account. *Psychological Medicine, 11,* 115–129.

Wirt, R. D., Lachar, D., Klinedinst, J. K., & Seat, P. D. (1977). *Multidimensional description of child personality: A manual for the Personality Inventory for Children.* Los Angeles: Western Psychological Services.

Zimmerman, I. L., & Allebrand, G. N. (1965). Personality characteristics and attitudes toward achievement of good and poor readers. *Journal of Educational Research, 57,* 28–30.

Index

J. A. Doane